M000252014

Shyam Singha studied osteopathy in London before qualifying as a doctor of acupuncture in Hong Kong and Taiwan. On his return to London, he set up the first premises for the British School of Acupuncture. He has also lived and studied with monks in the Gobi Desert, which is where he gained his insights into nutritional healing.

Alice Ebner
43161 Gatwick Sq.
Ashburn, VA 20147-4431

by the same author
Songs of Two Decades, 1962–1986

The
SECRETS
of NATURAL
HEALTH

Shyam Singha

ELEMENT
Shaftesbury, Dorset ● Boston, Massachusetts
Melbourne, Victoria

© Element Books Limited 1997
Text © Dr Shyam Singha 1997

First published in 1997 by
Element Books Limited

This revised edition published
in the UK in 1998 by
Element Books Limited
Shaftesbury, Dorset SP7 8BP

Published in the USA in 1998 by
Element Books, Inc.
160 North Washington Street, Boston, MA 02114

Published in Australia in 1998 by
Element Books
and distributed by Penguin Australia Limited
487 Maroondah Highway, Ringwood, Victoria 3134

All rights reserved.
No part of this book may be reproduced or utilized
in any form or by any means, electronic or mechanical,
without prior permission in writing from the Publisher.

Cover design by The Bridgewater Book Company
Designed and typeset by Linda Reed and Joss Nizan
Printed and bound in Great Britain by Creative Print
and Design (Wales), Ebbw Vale

British Library Cataloguing in Publication
data available

Library of Congress Cataloging in Publication
data available

ISBN 1–85230–938–5

Note from the publisher
Any information given in this book is not intended to be taken
as a replacement for medical advice. Any person with a condition
requiring medical attention should consult a qualified medical
practitioner or suitable therapist.

Contents

APPENDICES

ACKNOWLEDGEMENTS

For a generation of people who have attended Dr Shyam Singha's workshops or clinics, his words have become the gospel of Natural Health.

Since most of Shyam's time is taken up with the practical work of healing he has little time to write about the subject. The publishers are therefore pleased to rectify this omission by offering a comprehensive book of Shyam's work, authorized and checked by him.

This compilation – based on Shyam's seminars and discourses and individual meetings with him – has taken several years of dedicated work by **Sangitama Marion Huebner**, to whom the publishers express their thanks. She would like to give special thanks to Veeresh Denny Yuson, who inspired her to take on the compilation; the Humaniversity in the Netherlands for giving her the love, time and attention to make it happen; Bavala, Premdip and Sanman, who assisted with proofreading; and Bahulya for typing the manuscript.

The publishers are grateful to **Gregory van Dyk Watson** for skilfully adapting the material into book form.

Foreword

It was a great privilege to be asked to introduce this long-awaited book by Dr Shyam Singha. I have known him since I was a child through his association with my late father, another eminent holistic physician. Dr Singha's teachings have been passed on to me and used to a great extent in my own practice. For the student to be asked to comment on the master's techniques, it is indeed a privilege.

I believe that, finally, a self-help book has come forward that gives clear, practical advice on health from the perspective of Eastern philosophy, in a language that suits the West. So many books on health care direct us to specific products or techniques that, to some extent, disempower us – distancing us from our ability to heal ourselves. This book reverses the trend, allowing us to find our own therapies – often from ingredients in our own kitchens and gardens. At the same time Dr Singha explains and steers us through the practicalities of mind/body medicine.

The combination of nutritional advice and Ayurvedic food treatments with exercise and psychological techniques (derived from thousands of years of Ayurveda and decades of Dr Singha's personal experience) is unique and invaluable.

Part I introduces us to diet and general health care, while Parts II and III deal with common conditions and food sources. This book will be of value to individuals and their families as well as to professionals who will be able to integrate these simple but effective techniques into their practice – of both complementary and orthodox medicine.

Dr Shyam Singha's humour and enthusiasm are evident throughout, particularly in the 'Did you know?' sections where, in many cases, despite a lifetime involved with holistic health, I did not!

Read the book, keep it with your medicine chest and buy a copy for your primary health care practitioner. And with Dr Shyam Singha's help, stay happy and healthy.

Dr Rajendra Sharma

Introduction

Good health can be achieved by each and every one of us. And the means to achieve it lie within each person, rather than in global remedies and panaceas which, in my view, are dangerous and threaten our collective good health. In so far as each of us has a different constitution, remedies must always be related to individual human beings, adjusted to match each physiology and psychology.

Good health is natural and unique to each person. It involves listening to our bodies. Once we learn this art, many illnesses can be overcome by allowing the body to heal and rebalance itself without resorting to drugs and chemicals, which can cause more harm to the body in the long term and could well be the primary cause of the breakdown of our immune systems.

My purpose in writing this book is to pass on to you information that is in danger of becoming lost in this age of factory-processed foods – information that we should have learnt from our mothers and that should be part of our common folk memory. It is important to know that ordinary food and herbs eaten in a specific and balanced way can help you overcome a range of disorders as well as keep you healthy.

The information presented here is based on a number of lectures given by me over many years. I believe it contributes to our understanding of the body as a system. Nevertheless, I would like to emphasize that it is always preferable to consult an experienced healer for a definitive understanding of your health condition. It requires experience to understand the origin and nature of your ailments. Your body balance can change from month to month and even from week to week. An experienced healer can usually make a 'better diagnosis' of your unique constitution than you can yourself.

Good health is a matter of balance, both in the way we live and the food we eat. To be healthy involves knowing what steps to take and which foods to eat to rapidly restore this balance. And since each of us has a slightly different constitution, the remedy to restore us to good health will be slightly different. We need to discover for ourselves which remedy suits us best.

The Western approach persuades us that one specific remedy can be applied to a given symptom regardless of the individual and specific causes, which can be different for each person. This approach also induces us to be insensitive to our bodies, to ignore the first signs of discomfort and imbalance. And then, when it is almost too late, we willingly subject ourselves to a massive dose of Western-style drugs to deal with the symptoms. It's like ignoring the first signs that our car is not running properly, waiting instead until it finally breaks down at some inconvenient time and then having to pay a huge bill for the repair. A little preventative medicine to rectify the disorder would not only have been far more convenient but would also have saved us from a large subsequent bill.

In the same way, a more considered approach to health would save us from the damage of the side-effects of 'modern' medicine. We can help to avoid this by becoming aware of any mild disorders at an early stage and practising some simple preventative medicine, and by learning which commonly available foods or simple remedies can supply corrective treatment.

This book takes a tripartite view. Firstly, in Part I (The Diet Book) I show which foods and other remedies address nine of the basic body systems that govern our health. Secondly, in Part II (Health Manual) I describe a number of simple remedies for a range of common ailments, presented alphabetically from acne to wrinkles. Finally, in Part III (Food as Medicine) I explain the healing qualities of commonly available herbs and food sources, from alfalfa to yams.

The emphasis of this book is food as medicine. This naturally involves the whole human being. It is not helpful to simply address symptoms and not seek their underlying cause. The consequences of ignoring the actual cause of discomfort can often lead to unnecessary visits to specialists, who tend to treat symptoms rather than the person.

I often tell the seemingly silly story of a man whose eyes bulged and who experienced difficulty breathing when walking. A succession of doctors prescribed a range of remedies, from indigestion tablets to the removal of a number of organs, including his gall bladder and appendix.

With each successive treatment or organ removal the pain moved to different parts of his body, and in particular to his lower abdomen. Eventually a senior medical specialist evaluated his case and recommended a holiday on the basis that medical science had done all it could for him. Preparing to take a six-month holiday, the man visited his tailor to purchase new shirts and a suit. As the tailor called out the measurements, 'Collar fifteen-and-a-half,' the man interjected 'No, fourteen-and-a-half. I have been wearing a fourteen-and-a-half collar for the last fifteen years.' 'Sir,' replied the tailor, 'if you wear a fourteen-and-a-half collar, your eyes will bulge, you will experience difficulty in breathing and your lower abdomen will feel the strain when you walk.'

The mind has a greater impact on physical health than is often fully realized. Grounded in our subconscious are numerous cultural ideas about good, bad, right, wrong, moral and immoral. I acknowledge that these values act to an extent as the social glue which holds together the fabric of civilization, but – where these values are negative and bigoted – as individuals we pay an almighty price.

Sexual taboos, for instance, create unnatural social attitudes. They result in confusion between sex and love, superficiality in ordinary social encounters, and the distortion of *romance*. Only a sexually confused society produces romance, replacing naturalness with fantasy. Evidence of this distortion can be seen in the way that sex is used to market consumer products – such as car tyres – that possess no ostensible connection with sex. The worst result of negative attitudes to sexuality is repression. One of the consequences is sexual crime, which seems to mystify the very people – such as Church and political leaders – who are themselves responsible for having compounded and perpetuated the problem.

Our principal way to counteract these negative influences is by using our *will* to realize the truth, by meditation and by depolarizing the negativity. By dispersing negativity we can retain our natural instincts (*hara*) and our ability to make authentic choices.

In the positively oriented person the energy flow (*kundalini*) in the body is upward. It circulates through the seven energy centres (*chakras*) in our body. This flow is generated in the sex or root centres (perineum area) and moves through the gut centre, the solar plexus, the heart centre, the throat centre and the mouth centre to the 'third eye'. In the sex-obsessed person the energy flow is downward. Such a person will experience a depletion of energy if this flow is not eventually counter-balanced.

The two opposing energies, *yin* and *yang*, can be used beneficially in *tantra*, an Eastern movement that applies its understanding of the kundalini to good effect. It enables men and women to meet sexually with heightened sensitivity. The resultant cosmic energy of such a union *resolves* rather than *dissolves* the differences between men and women. Such a union is as natural as that of the wind (yin) and the sky (yang).

Uniforms of the mind

Given the prevailing social climate, it is hardly surprising that so many people seek refuge in fixed belief systems. I refer to these rigid attitudes as *uniforms of the mind*. Their negative impact upon our health is greater than we realize. Uniforms of the mind come in the guise of dogma, duty, ideas of God, country, class, hierarchy, club, school, profession, the right side of the railway track.

In most cases the adoption of a mind-uniform is an attempt to find meaning. But meaning is specific and personal, with value only to the adopter. People will sacrifice themselves for a meaning, even to the point of martyrdom in some cases. In the hands of the malevolent, uniforms can become cudgels of authority – army fatigues, religious robes and police blue being the most obvious. In saying this I do not mean to malign the many good people who wear uniforms. I am referring to more than actual uniforms. I am referring to the way in which we adopt a particular way of thinking and behaving when we don a specific role, usually a job role. The role itself tends to extend and circumscribe simultaneously our span of authority. This is most visible, as I'm sure we've all noticed, when a person takes on a new job and amends his or her personality to suit the job role, almost unthinkingly. When we adopt the mannerisms of the role, the uniform to which I refer takes shape. Whether policeman, doctor, priest, banker, salesman, army officer, pop musician, professor or entrepreneur, we automatically think of a particular personality style, together with matching clothes. We become the role that we play. And in so doing we risk losing our very uniqueness as we cut the cloth of our personality to suit the role that we adopt. While we achieve a sense of security in merging with a group identity, we pay a price – reflected in our mental, physical and spiritual health – that is not always immediately evident.

To the extent that mind-uniforms induce people to adopt postures (mental, physical and emotional) that are divergent from their essential nature, they are antithetical to good health. The more mind-maps that we hold about ourselves and other people, the more we endeavour to fit ourselves and others into them. These mental maps detract from our ability to engage with people in a unique and open-minded manner and to hear what they are really saying to us beyond their actual words. And yet we all ascribe to the truism that no two people are identical.

In the same way that our presumptions hamper our understanding of other people, they also stand in the way of our experience of our own bodies and hamper our ability to hear what our bodies are really saying to us. To overcome this we need to engage with life in a way that goes beyond the limited ability of the mind.

Healing

Healing is the birthright of the body. However, healing can be hindered by doctors, surgeons, pills, exercise fanatics, colonic irrigators and many others who believe in quick cures. The body has an almost infinite ability to heal and regenerate itself. Many Eastern traditions attribute this ability to a primordial energy known as *chi* or *prana*. Although inherent in the body from birth, this energy can be systematically suppressed by various types of drugs, antibiotics, painkillers and muscle relaxants. While these remedies may help us to some extent in the short term, they also interfere with the body's own healing process.

The net result is that we suffer more illness from bad living habits than from actual disease. The pressures upon us in modern society are so great that we are more prone to stress-related ailments than probably any other kind of illness. Stress subdues our basic energy and prevents the body from performing the job of healing. Healing requires time. However, the fast-food era encourages us to want everything to happen instantly. This leads inexorably to our use of instant solutions such as pain-killers, anti-inflammatants, acid reducers, sleep inducers, uppers, downers and so forth. We want to suppress the cause and vaporize the symptoms. We thereby avoid facing the fact that the cause of illness lies within each individual. Until we deal directly with the cause, and until it is overcome, the dis-ease and discomfort will remain to haunt us in a variety of different manifestations. There are, however, ways to discover the causes of our illnesses, many of which have been known since ancient times. One of these is *ayurveda* (self-knowledge).

Ayurveda

Ayurveda encompasses not only science but also philosophy, religion and specific techniques for living well. 'Philosophy' is used here to mean love of truth and truth as being (pure existence), and 'religion' in the sense that one becomes a witness of oneself. Ayurveda states that every individual is a unique phenomenon and indivisible from the cosmos. Whatever exists in the macrocosm, exists also in the microcosm. Every individual is a manifestation of cosmic consciousness.

The healing science of ayurveda is based on the total understanding of the individual constitution. Every individual must first get to know his own constitution. He is required to find out what kind of diet and lifestyle best suits him. Every individual is composed of mind, body and spirit; although the philosophy of each element is identical, its manifestation will differ according to emphasis. Hence ayurveda, from its concern with the physical basis of life, induces harmony of mind and spirit. To encourage this, ayurveda recommends taking up some form of yoga, which teaches control of the body and mind, and their harmonization with spirit. In its widest sense, ayurveda teaches how to use the mind to balance the demands of body and spirit. The aim is to reach a balance called health or *svastha*, from *sva* (self) and *stha* (established). While most of this book deals with the selection of certain foods in order to overcome specific disorders, it is also a statement of the ayurvedic approach.

Western physicians tend to work with named diagnoses and their infectious causes, rather than with the whole person. They tend to specialize in particular organs of the body such as the liver, lungs or heart. Western medicine's ability to fire a bullet-pill at the bull's-eye of a disease, or simply to remove or replace a failing organ, is much admired as one of the hallmarks of progress, but it encourages medical people to target symptoms rather than causes. As a consequence people are encouraged to live to excess and ignore discomfort until it becomes a veritable disease. The disease is thereafter treated while the body's natural gift for self-healing is ignored.

In ayurveda we learn about the relationship between self and universe. The ancient Rishis (Hindu sages) realized that human consciousness is a fragment of nature's own consciousness. This insight identifies different forms of 'I', the individual self. The 'I' is expressed in waves of kinetic energy, in material particles of potential energy and in subjective consciousness. In Sanskrit, these are called respectively, *rajas*, *tamas* and *sattva*. Rajas is activity, tamas inertia, and sattva the balancer of both. Collectively, these three are called *gunas*. They control the five great elements of our body. By working with these elements we can influence the regulation of the metabolic functions of the body.

Healing can also be effected by something as simple as the laying on of hands. Such a phenomenon has been with us for centuries. This happens when a person who is centred induces peace and serenity in another and allows that person to relax and let go, so that the body can take over its own healing work unhindered by outside influences, whether they be chemical or otherwise. When the head is emptied of extraneous influences, heart and *hara* (instincts) come into play, and the healing process starts, mostly by simply acknowledging our own personality and structure. However, it is often necessary to go through major changes to get back to who we really are.

Some obvious exceptions to this general rule are epidemics, food poisoning, catastrophes and car accidents. In these instances we must also consider the external and internal hygiene needed to maintain the status quo if foreign invaders of any kind have been the cause of the dis-equilibrium, dis-comfort or dis-ease. *It is important to note that ayurveda does not provide cures as such; rather, it aids to enable the body to heal itself.*

Let me provide an example. One of my patients was a priest with a 12-year history of stomach problems. Medication, diet, meditation, fasting, pills and potions did not seem to work. Then one day while he was lying on the treatment couch, I asked him, 'What can't you stomach?' His reply was slow, meek, but genuine: 'Being a priest', he said. 'What would you like to be?' was my next question. 'An antiques restorer.' 'Then why the blazes don't you?' I shouted. 'I can't, I can't,' he cried. Both his father and his grandfather before him were priests. They wanted him to continue the tradition, so he became a priest, but his desire to be an antiques restorer never left him. I told him to leave the country and go somewhere where nobody knew him and start a small business as an antiques restorer. He complained about his obligations to his parishioners, his wife and his two sons, to name but a few. I asked him what would happen if he died of a bad stomach ulcer or Crohn's disease or some other malady. Eventually I persuaded him, and he went. Three years later his wife and children joined him. One day he telephoned me to announce how happy he now was. He wanted me to visit him so that I could see for myself what he had accomplished as a result of my good advice. Instead I told him that his task was unfinished and that there was something else that was required of him. I told him to stand in a specific place in the town and tell bible stories to the people who gathered around him. He was astonished. I explained that now that he was open, content, satisfied and truthful, his stories would contain meaning that was previously lacking; up to the time that he left his parish, his stories had been scripturally appropriate but lacking in emotional truth. A year later I received another telephone call. He wanted me to visit him in order to see how many people gathered to listen to his stories. Although this was a unique response to a unique situation, the principle can be applied to the situation many people find themselves in.

Of course, if we can never generalize, there would be no education, culture, science, history, mathematics, art, religion, codes of etiquette, laws, rules, or even the literature, to teach us how to deal with unique situations. There would be total chaos, whereas now at least we live in controlled chaos. This is demonstrated in the Western approach to medicine. Yet despite the differences in application, the same principles apply to modern medicine as apply to ayurveda or any other ancient system. Let us now look at three vital factors in all physical healing.

Cleansing, nourishing and balancing

When something is blocked, you need to unblock it. When something is undernourished, you must nourish it. And then, after unblocking/cleansing and nourishing, you have to attain balance. In balance there is no dis-ease. You may achieve that balance through osteopathy and chiropractic, by altering your diet, by paying attention to your psyche and spirit, and by shouting, teasing and laughing. Other methods, such as the Alexander technique, which are primarily concerned with balance are also useful. In balance there is no absolute. There is yin and there is yang. Both are present.

Nothing should be taken for granted, whether it be medicines, relationships, God or the wind. If you do, you make a big error. It is only man that wants to create constancy and certainty. In so far as man succeeds in creating a sense of permanence, he becomes fixed. He ends up being controlled by all the fixtures and fixities he has created. Consequently he ends up locked in a prison of his own making. The mystic, Gurdjieff, used to say: 'Unless you have realized that you are in a prison, there is no way that you will come out of it.' When this awareness dawns upon a person, it is usually a sudden realization.

One day I received a new patient who had been diagnosed as having cancer. After he had explained that he was vegetarian and went to the temple every day, I asked him about the nature of his work. His retort was, 'Why do you ask that? What does that have to do with the cancer?' I discovered that he was a money lender, someone who charged vast amounts of interest to people who often could not afford it. I asked him how many people he might have met and if they responded to him in a way that provided him with healing and nourishing energy. Of course they did not. As a consequence of his activities, many houses were destroyed, many lives were fractured, and there was much unhappiness. Those people who were affected by his activities were sending him negative vibrations which caused his illness. I told him that I could not help him. As soon as realization struck him, there was a short remission. Instead of dying in three months, he died in three years. So, at least he had time to repent and come to terms with himself and his life. Injury to others is paid back to us in various ways: 'what goes around comes around.'

There are no quick remedies for achieving balance, such as fasting to compensate for years of unhealthy living. You can fast for six weeks and feel good. The next moment your sense of wellbeing can be reversed. When you are fasting, you may be thinking of the feast to come. Alternatively, when you are feasting, you may be saying to yourself: 'Don't worry, tomorrow I will fast.' Both are illusions for which you may pay dearly.

Is it medicine that makes you better?

From time immemorial mankind has searched for a panacea, a secret formula or ambrosia which would not only bring relief from illness but provide longevity, eternal youth, strength and stamina.

There are many stories of old potions – Chinese, Egyptian, Greek, Indian and American Indian. Desperately ill people always seek the unknown, because the known has either not worked or has had too many side-effects. And if they are not looking for secret potions, they are seeking out disciplines. But neither school, Occidental or Oriental, can provide what is not there or act as a panacea. The Occidental school promises relief with prescriptions, whereas the Oriental school promises relief if you change your style of living. Both have their side-affects, some serious some not. If you become macrobiotic without much heed, just as a fad, you may become depleted. If you overdose yourself with pain killers you may be deleted, literally.

The old way of medication was to make the body strong by purging it of debris, old blood and toxins, and feeding it with nutritious food. The modern way does not worry about food at all. Its sole concern is the pathogen, such as bacteria and viruses. It wants to kill these bacteria somehow, even though it means harming the host also. It very often happens that the bacteria, when subdued by a drug, mutate and change and return in a more virulent manner than before, giving altogether different symptoms to different parts of the body. The physician can logically say, 'We tackled the last one all right; we shall tackle this one with a different style of attack.' In the end, chronic disease increases and the resistance of the body is lowered to the extent that people become invalids, living the rest of their lives depending on compensatory pills and potions, bearing more and more operation scars.

Is it healthy to be unique?

From the time we are born, most of the simple decisions are taken away from us. We are constantly told what to do and what not to do. In childhood, how often have we not at some stage heard, 'Eat your dinner *now*, because it's dinner time. If you don't eat it now, don't ask for food later when you're hungry.' These experiences mould the child into the ways of society rather than allowing it to grow up relatively free from social constraints. The mealtime example serves to underline the conditions under which children are born and bred to conform to the ways of society and the group. By its very nature society is inherently hostile to individuality. It has an inbuilt resistance to allowing the individual to flower in his or her own way.

All social institutions, whether medical, religious, social or economic, demand a high degree of mental conformity as the price of membership. By the age of around seven most children are already indoctrinated into a conformist mode. Whilst there are certainly advantages to social conformity, there is also a price that is not immediately apparent. In internalizing and adopting society's conceptual models and structures, the individual is induced into acting in violation of his own nature.

Society conditions us to such an extent that we tend to conform not only in the way that we think, but also in the way that we live, especially with regard to eating habits. Instead of discovering our uniqueness and living according to our own inner dictates, most of us follow instead the dictates of parents, politicians, clergy, the media and peer groups. In obeying these external voices – which may even be the original cause of some of our worst illnesses – we deny our essential nature.

Intellect and intelligence in health

An analogy for the ayurvedic way of healing is that it is similar to listening to somebody playing a tune, such as a Bach 'Partita', or 'Singing in the Rain'. Whichever instrument is used – flute, banjo, piano, saxophone, mouth-organ or the human voice – the tune remains the same. Ayurveda is about recognizing the tune, and for this we may need our senses rather than our intellectual function.

It is a difficult matter to define health. Health is a symphony. If we are in harmony, we are healthy; but when there is discord, we become aware that something is wrong. When health is flowing, we tend not to think about the organs of the body; we only think about them when they fail to function.

It is almost an assumption in ayurvedic healing that when the mind becomes over-dominant, the body falls ill. Although the mind is the container of much information, it is not the possessor of real knowledge. It deals mainly with collected data and information. It can be likened to watching a cricket match; we are not the players, merely the spectators. The mind is an instrument for observing and collecting; it has no fundamental intelligence. Intelligence in the sense to which I am referring provides a deeper and more fundamental understanding than the mind.

Intelligence is the original Buddhahood. Intelligence is our own consciousness. It is our own centre. The intellect is somewhat superficial by comparison with the intelligence that is intuitive and can sense the instincts (the *hara*). This kind of intelligence always touches the centre of our being, which many of us have forgotten.

The mind is also a dissipater. It tends to destroy rather than increase energy. When the mind is worried and anxious, the body produces acid. Sadly, worrying about anxiety rarely redresses the situation. When a bus or a train is ten minutes late, we often become anxious. When we hold our breath or become angry, our mouth becomes dry and our body produces more acid; our bile is increased and our energy is sapped. These symptoms are often the result of anxiety generated by the mind.

Meditation

Meditating creates a colossal amount of energy. Meditating can stop the mind from dissipating its energy by enabling it to accumulate energy in silence. When we are not dissipating our energy with mental chattering and become centred, we can generate a fountain of energy. Real consciousness only begins when the mind stops chattering. We then become conscious, alive, here and in the present. Most forms of meditation – Sufi dancing, fasting, and many other methods – allow us, for a moment, to become conscious. These are the same roads that have taken people to superconscious enlightenment, and even to a state of collective superconsciousness. I believe that this is what both Christ and Buddha felt. Beyond that is cosmic consciousness, the beautiful source where everything has been written. However, most of the time we are too busy with our need for ego gratification to experience what it offers. It's so simple and beautiful, like a seed, a plant, a little flower with its essence travelling upwards. So simple.

Meditation is not a system. If you want to make a start, do what feels harmonious. Harmony means music with which you are in tune. Meditation is a way to link with and communicate with our inner being – each time afresh.

Different disciplines are available. Try to discover what sort of meditation suits you best – it is not the same as praying. Transcendental, Zazen, Sufi Whirling, Hatha Yoga, Mantric, Yantric and Tantric are just a few of the numerous methods and practices. Once you are ready, the right form will discover you. Trust your intuition.

Disease

Finally we can talk about disease. When the body tells you, 'I experience discomfort,' it will become disease if you fail to listen. The important lesson is to learn to 'catch it early'.

1st stage: dis-ease/discomfort
2nd stage: disease – label, name
3rd stage: the suppression or expression of it

Our tendency is to suppress what the body is saying, with or without drugs. Although we may take aspirin or paracetamol for a headache, the headache is still there even though we no longer feel it. If the condition is suppressed rather than expressed, it may become inflammation or eventually an 'itis': appendicitis, colitis, cystitis. 'Itis' means inflammation. Thereafter more drastic measures are called for, such as operations to remove tonsils, appendix, kidney stones or gall bladder. But surgical intervention does not necessarily remove the cause of an illness or condition. There are more gentle ways to help the body help itself. We can also treat a disease by increasing the energy of the body so that it can heal itself – by treating the body from the inside out instead of from the outside in.

We can use herbs, diets, homoeopathy, acupuncture, water cures (such as mineral, mud or sitz baths) and fasting. None of these produces dangerous or unpleasant side-effects. All chemical therapy, without exception, produces some side-effect for which there is often no remedy, as in the case of chemotherapy.

What is health?

In general, health is a lack of discomfort – physical, mental, spiritual, psychological and economic – combined with an essential and balanced degree of tension to ensure that we are not completely inert. Wellbeing is an experience which we are all aware of when it is present.

Good health, however, requires that we regularly maintain our bodies and monitor our lives. This book deals primarily with the ingestion of the right foods to promote good health. To complement my message I also want to stress that much of 'good health' is achieved by a mixture of common sense and a balanced approach to life. It entails listening to our bodies. A balanced approach involves viewing our discomforts in a whole way rather than as a specific and particular set of symptoms. For example, a lung problem can lead to overheating and itching, followed by scratching and eczema. To treat the eczema is to treat the symptom, whereas by looking at the lung problem we might find that the person is holding his breath and unwittingly not exhaling properly. If we delve further, we might find that holding his breath is a response to a given set of circumstances in his life.

Nutrition

Nutrition is not generally regarded as a solution to ailments. It is easier for medical doctors to prescribe medicines and treatments that reflect the orientation of their training. Their tendency is to respond to illnesses by focusing on the pathology and by using surgical, antibiotic or antiviral methods. The initial symptom may or may not subside, but in the meantime it might produce three or four other symptoms. This is one of the maladies of our society.

While I am not advocating the non-use of medication, I am strongly against the unnecessary, continuous and repetitive use of medication without regular evaluation. Many ailments are caused by ill-conceived thoughts, an inappropriate lifestyle and bad eating habits. It is an old truism that 'we are what we eat'.

In this book I offer a few solutions and suggestions that have been successfully prescribed to my patients over many years of practice. It is my hope that you may, in this increasingly complex and technical world, find some of these simple remedies of some benefit.

PART I

THE DIET BOOK

Diets for different purposes

CHAPTER 1

The Biological System

Before suggesting any diets to remedy defects in the biological system, I will describe the manner in which it functions and the way in which it can be impacted psychologically.

The biological system is a process of ingestion, digestion, assimilation and elimination. Fundamentally the body is like a tube: nutrition enters through the mouth, travels via the oesophagus into the stomach, from the stomach through the pylorus into the duodenum, and from the duodenum, through the jejunum and the ileum to the iliocaecal valve. From there the remaining solids pass into the colon and exit via the rectum. This process is the job of the body tube.

We need therefore to ensure that this body tube and its organs are capable of ingesting efficiently. Food needs to be well chewed to facilitate digestion by the body. When food is inappropriately mixed or taken at irregular intervals, or if you are highly stressed, the system is unable to properly digest it.

Pre-digestion takes place between the mouth and the pylorus, the last part of the stomach. Actual digestion occurs between the pylorus, duodenum and jejunum. In the duodenum the pancreatic juices and gall bladder juices are added. The stomach is totally acidic. The acidity of the stomach has to be converted and the pH has to be balanced to a normal level of around 7.0. Thereafter digestion starts to take place.

Food is assimilated through the villi of the small intestines. The villi are numerous little hairs through which the fructose and glucose are assimilated. It is here that fats are changed to lipase, protinase and amino acids, and starches changed to glucose.

All foods, excluding vitamins, minerals and trace elements, have the capability of being converted into glucose – fuel for the body. The nutrients are assembled in the small intestines, from where they are transported by the hepatic vein to the liver. The liver purifies the nutrients. An excess of sugar in the blood is converted into glycogen and deposited. In this way the body maintains its balance.

Glucose is released via the liver into the vena cava, from where the blood and the nutrients are transported to the lungs. The lungs oxygenate the blood, which then goes directly to the heart. The heart in turn pumps the blood through the aorta and on to the kidneys. This process is both simple and yet miraculous. It functions automatically and continuously without conscious intervention.

Psychology of digestion

Our state of mind and emotional balance are critical at meal times because they determine the extent to which we digest our food. In order for the nutrients contained in the food to be absorbed by the body they need to be properly assimilated. If the nutrients are not assimilated, the food will pass through the body and be eliminated without any benefit to the body. In many cases we would have been better off had we not eaten at all. It is remarkable that we are still alive in view of the ways in which some of us abuse our bodies.

Our thoughts when we sit down to eat have a fundamental effect on our digestion. As an experiment, think of some of your favourite foods and notice how you feel and what takes place in your mouth and your stomach. Now think of your least favourite food and notice your feelings and the sensations in your stomach. Possibly you began to salivate when you thought of your favourite food. The juices generated by our thoughts determine how thoroughly the food is broken down in the stomach and assimilated.

It is important therefore to ensure that your state of mind at mealtimes is conducive to digestion. If not, you may just as well throw away the food for all the benefit that you are likely to receive. How you eat the food is almost as important as what you eat. Often, remedies are required to compensate for not having absorbed the nutrients from the food we have eaten.

My recommendation is that when sitting down to eat, ensure firstly that you are actually hungry and not simply proposing to eat because it is a certain time of day. Next, meditate, or put yourself into a relaxed state of being that will facilitate food intake. Use mealtimes as occasions to take time out for yourself. Be kind to yourself and to your body at these times. Treat them as your sacred moments during the day.

My general guidelines for choice of diet are:

1 Choose your diet carefully: vegetarian or non-vegetarian.
2 Follow your intuition – don't force yourself.
3 Follow what pleases your palate.

✳ Juice fast

Before starting the fast, attune your body by eating only raw fruit for 1–2 days.

A fast for 3 days will give the body a basic cleansing. Consult your healing practitioner if you plan to conduct a lengthy fast as problems can occur. Constipation, emotional upsets, skin irritations and headaches are all signs of the cleansing process at work. However, it is best to seek expert advice.

A 10-day fast will bring relief from most complaints, but you can continue it for up to 3 weeks if necessary. If you are taking homoeopathic drops it is usually advisable to continue the treatment. But you can stop taking vitamins and start again after the fast. Remember – always check with your healing practitioner. It is normal to keep working during a fast, but be careful not to over-reach yourself. You will need time for your assignments (see below), extra sleep and meditation. Winter is a time when the body stores rather than cleanses. Springtime and late summer are ideal for your annual body cleansing.

If you suffer from any severe disease, you need to check with your health practitioner whether a fast or diet would be beneficial for you. People with heart problems are definitely advised *not* to go on a fast without professional supervision.

Daily schedule

8.00   Juice of a whole lemon in a glass of boiled water, hot or cold.

10.00   Orange juice diluted in water.

12.00   Grapefruit juice with 1 tablespoon of psyllium husks added.

14.00   Place 500g of green grapes (the common variety and the cheapest obtainable) in a piece of muslin and squeeze into a tumbler. Pour one third of the resultant juice into a glass of hot or cold boiled water. Drink 3 cups.

16.00   Squeeze the juice from 5–6 tomatoes into a tumbler of hot or cold boiled water.

18.00   Same as 8.00.

20.00   Same as 10.00.

Whenever you break your fast, make a concoction from fresh vegetables such as a scrubbed carrot, a potato, some celery, watercress, a tomato, an onion and any other vegetables that you can find. Place them in 1 litre of cold water, then boil down to 500ml. Strain the liquid off and drink very slowly with a piece of dry toast.

Some tips

All fruit juices and vegetables have a cleansing effect due to their high content of minerals and vitamins and the absence of starches and toxins. Read about the specific fruit or vegetable in Part II, Food as Medicine.

You can drink as much cold boiled water as you require in between the above times and it is also permissible to have a slippery elm malted drink once a day.

While on a juice diet or a fast, relax and do a lot of deep breathing. Deep breathing helps not only to oxygenate the blood, but also to relax the abdominal muscles. Abdominal massages and foot reflex massages for the lungs and colon are also very beneficial during fasting.

If you find your mouth becomes murky and the tongue coated, take some raw lemon juice, place it in an eggcup with approximately 2 teaspoons of warm water and immerse your tongue in the solution for a few seconds. Then scrape the tongue with a spoon. Gargle with the remainder of the solution and spit it out.

Do not chew gum: your body will receive a signal to produce digestive enzymes and will become confused when no food arrives.

It is also important to sip fluids slowly rather than gulping them down. Juices and broths should be sipped only. Eat the fluids and drink the solids!

Assignments

1 During the fast, take a long walk of some 3 or 4km.
2 In the morning use a dry brush to stimulate the skin and increase the circulation, always remembering to brush towards the heart.
3 Take a lukewarm bath at night to induce sound sleep.

❈ Three-day fast and cleanse

Daily schedule

8.15 750ml of mineral water.
9.00 750ml of mineral water.
10.00 Weak green China tea or dandelion coffee.
13.00 Juice of an orange in a glass of hot water.
16.00 Juice of an orange in a glass of hot water, or a cup of green vegetable water (made by simmering various root and green vegetables in water for about half an hour).
19.00 Same as 16.00.
21.00 Same as 16.00.

On the third day drink the juice of 3 apples at 17.00 and of about 200g grapes at 18.00.

At the end of the fast, avoid greasy food, meat, cheese and beans to begin with. Eat only salads and fruit, crackers, or grains such as rice, millet, buckwheat. Chew every morsel slowly to avoid overeating.

Enemas

If you lack roughage and fibre in your diet, and are imbibing only juices and broth, the bowels become inactive and can stop working. An enema in these circumstances may be helpful – but not always! If after three days on a fast, you have not had a bowel movement, try a *coffee enema* (see Appendix B). This is very stimulating and cleansing. One enema is enough to clean the colon. Do not repeat once movement is restored to the bowels. Prolonged constipation will eventually cause auto-intoxication as the colon reabsorbs accumulated toxins. In general, thin people tend not to require enemas because their systems are usually very 'airy' and not stagnant. Conversely, people with more generous amounts of body fat are more likely to require an enema since excess fat tends to imply a more sluggish system.

RECIPES
See Appendix B for coffee enema, or take 1 tablespoon olive oil in 750ml lukewarm water. If you suffer from excess toxicity make an enema from comfrey tea.

❋ Grape diet

This diet is helpful with the following indications:
- intestinal putrefactions, constipation
- cardiac affections
- gastro-intestinal catarrh
- chronic bronchitis
- emphysema
- scrofula
- enlargement of the spleen
- chronic cystitis
- gout
- dyspepsia
- melancholy and spleen (changing moods)
- obesity
- indigestion
- liver complaints and hepatic disorders
- Bright's disease
- biliousness
- gastritis
- anaemia
- rheumatism
- kidney complaints and nephritis

Grapes are very nourishing. They are rich in elements and minerals such as potassium, sodium, calcium, magnesium, iron, phosphates, sulphates, chlorine and fructose and have an amazing ability to rebuild tissue. A number of unconfirmed post-war stories in Europe relate that the wounds of soldiers with no food other than grapes, healed faster than those of other soldiers.

A popular diet in the grape cure institutions of Europe for the treatment of various chronic disorders involves eating grapes for 3 days. On the first day the patient takes about 500g of grapes, increasing this amount by 500g daily until a maximum of 3kg per day is reached. No other food is allowed.

If you follow a grape cure for more than 7 days, it is recommended that you start by drinking only water for 1–2 days (no other food) until your body develops an appetite for the grapes. This diet cleanses the stomach and intestines. Prepare a schedule where you have a grape meal every 2 hours, remembering to chew the skin and seeds thoroughly.

Eat as many as 7 grape meals a day. During the first days constipation can occur because of an accumulation of grape seeds in the intestine; they may well block normal elimination. This will not happen, however, if you chew the seeds thoroughly. It is better to start with a small amount of grapes, 500g to 1½kg a day, gradually increasing to the maximum.

Special attention needs to be paid to the cleaning of the grapes, especially if they are your sole nutritional source. Most people do not realize that some pesticides are water-insoluble so that they can resist rain. The grapes can be rinsed in salt water for about 10 minutes, or in a 1 per cent solution of hydro-chloric acid (HCl) in water for 5 minutes. After this treatment rinse again with water. The salt/HCl solution is best kept in an earthenware container, and can be used for up to 1 week.

The grape cure is effective in the treatment of obesity. It cleanses the body by flushing out toxic waste. Vomiting, diarrhoea, fever, weakness and an urge to rest, headaches, migraines, backache and other body pains are symptoms of the cleansing process at work. If they occur, it is important to continue the diet while simultaneously listening to the needs of your body. A headache might suggest that you drink more hot water. Backache might make you aware of the tension in your body. Massage will generally provide relief in such circumstances.

It is important to emerge slowly from the diet and not to indulge in too large a variety of foods immediately afterwards. It is best to eat raw food for a few days, and gradually include cooked food in the evenings, together with some milk or bread. Eat cooked and uncooked food separately for a while.

Under medical supervision grapes are used for the treatment of various diseases and conditions such as cancer, tumours, pneumonic disorders, mental disease, nervous disorders, sexual problems, and diabetes. Grapes are strong blood purifiers and are used to detoxify the stomach and intestines. These more complicated grape cures are best conducted under medical supervision and with the support of an experienced healer.

❊ Grape and fruit diet

Another version of the grape diet involves eating between 500g and 1kg of grapes for breakfast and raw foods of any kind during the rest of the day. This is an excellent diet for constipation, auto-intoxication, and other chronic disorders.

A good way to conduct the fruit diet is to eat 2 oranges and an apple 3 times a day – or 2 oranges and a pear or a peach. Drink 6–8 glasses of water during the day. This diet may be continued for several days, up to a maximum of 3 weeks.

Acid and sub-acid fruits, when eaten ripe and uncooked, provide organic digestive chemicals similar to pepsin, which is needed to break down proteins. They also supply the active phosphorus compounds needed for the brain, nerve cells, the spinal cord, bone marrow and muscles. Acid fruits include lemons, pineapples, tangerines, oranges, grapefruit, limes, gooseberries, red currants, tomatoes, cranberries and some varieties of apples and strawberries. Lemons are highly acidic, and when baked, become sub-acid. A very sweet apple is sub-acid.

Through elimination we often lose minerals. Stomach cramps are a sign that this is happening. Acute cramps indicate a lack of sodium; if they are more consistent and dull, magnesium deficiency is usually the cause. *Tissue salts* such as magnesium phosphoricum D6 or magnesium sulfuricum will stop the cramps almost immediately. I can recommend Dr Schuessler's tissue salts (see p. 66).

For further cleansing make a drink from equal quantities of the following freshly made juices:

- watercress
- mustard cress
- spinach
- celery
- cucumber

Add sorrel or chives to taste. I suggest 1 cup, 3 times a day.

❋ Low-fat diet

The low-fat diet is ideal for people who are overweight – who are more prone than the less well-padded to develop kidney trouble, heart disease, diabetes, high blood pressure, psychological problems, liver damage and liver disease such as hepatitis. They also invariably have a high level of cholesterol in the blood. A low-fat diet is also recommended for people who show signs of hyperglycaemia.

High cholesterol levels

Fats should be avoided where possible – saturated and unsaturated. Saturated fats are found mainly in animal products. Cholesterol blood levels are raised by saturated fatty acids. Unsaturated fatty acids are found in vegetable fats. Two notable exceptions are cocoa oil and coconut oil, which are almost saturated. Heated vegetable oil and the fats in roasted nuts are saturated. Fish tends to have more unsaturated than saturated fats.

While it is true that unsaturated fats lower cholesterol levels in the blood, they create havoc by raising triglyceride levels. Over the long term a high consumption of fats in the human body leads to the following problems:

- capillary blockage
- depletion of vitamin E
- gallstones
- promotion of tumour growth

Also, fats provoke the production of bile acids, which in excess can lead to the growth of anaerobic bacteria, a carcinogenic environment.

All fats form a fatty film around elements in the blood – particularly the red blood cells – and prevent them from functioning properly. The effects can be felt instantly. Note how tired you feel after a meal that is rich in fats. This is because the body and the brain have failed to receive a sufficient supply of oxygen. It is by contrast possible to feel energized after a lighter and more balanced meal. When we eat fatty meals, the body burns glucose very quickly to force it to use the large fat reserves. A byproduct of burning fats is an acid-metabolite called ketones. Too many ketones in the body create a collapse – ketosis. A diet low in fats is thus the most beneficial.

Cholesterol is a sterol – like a wax – and does not dissolve in the blood plasma. The body needs a certain amount of cholesterol to make bile acids for digestion and steroid hormones such as progesterone and the adrenal glucocorticoids. It is also found in nerve fibre sheaths and cell membranes.

But an excess of cholesterol in the blood causes it to stick to artery walls, hardening and narrowing them. These deposits are especially dangerous in the coronary arteries. The more the plaque builds up, the more slowly the blood flows towards the heart. If the plaque builds up to such an extent that it effectively closes the blood vessel, the tissue dependent on the blood fed by that artery dies. When part of the heart begins to die, a myocardial infarct occurs. When a section of the brain is similarly starved, a stroke occurs.

Daily schedule

ON RISING

Have an eggcup of safflower oil (25ml) on an empty stomach. Then suck a slice of lemon.

BREAKFAST
Weak black tea, herbal or fruit tea – skimmed milk and sugar can be added if you wish.
Raw or stewed fruit.
Porridge or breakfast cereal with skimmed milk and sugar.
Boiled smoked haddock or white fish.
Brown bread toasted, with honey or syrup.

MID-MORNING
Glass of lemon barley water.

LUNCH
Boiled or steamed white fish, chicken, turkey, stewed liver or kidney, or very lean beef or mutton.
Potatoes, boiled or baked in jackets or mashed with skimmed milk.
Boiled vegetables – such as cabbage, cauliflower, spinach, celery, carrots, parsnips, turnips – or salad.
Boiled rice, skimmed milk pudding, stewed or fresh fruit.
Glass of lemon barley water.

TEA
Weak tea, herbal or fruit tea – skimmed milk and sugar are allowed.

DINNER
As lunch.

BEFORE RETIRING (and during the night if awake)
Glass of lemon barley water – hot or cold.

DO NOT EAT ANY OF THE FOLLOWING
Butter, cream, margarine, dripping, suet, lard, oil, mayonnaise, eggs – or any dishes containing these items. Fat fish such as salmon, herring, mackerel, bloaters, kippers. Duck, goose, foie gras. Fat meat, pork, ham, bacon, sausages. Fried foods. Roast potatoes, potato chips, fried onions. Yorkshire pudding, suet dumplings, crust and pies. Suet pudding, pastry, fritters, ice cream, cake mixture puddings, macaroni, cakes. Chocolate, cocoa flavourings. Whole milk. Chocolate, coffee, caramel, marzipan, nuts. Shortbread, biscuits containing fat.

Assignments

These may seem unusual, but consider performing them in the interests of your health.

1 Sing loudly for 10 minutes.
2 Skip with a rope for 10 minutes.
3 In the shower, run hot and cold water on the spine – 3 minutes hot and 1 minute cold. Do this 3 times and finish with a cold shower.
4 Have a tickling session with a partner for 10 minutes.
5 Eat an avocado, a papaya and a cos (Romaine) lettuce every day.

❋ Monofasts

In a monofast only one kind of fruit or vegetable is eaten. This both cleanses the body and allows the stomach to rest (because no proteins and fats are eaten, there is no requirement for hydrochloric acid and bile, which digest and emulsify these foods in the stomach). The body utilizes all that we eat in the form of glucose, and all fructose is changed to glucose by a relatively easy digestive process.

The best fasts are with plums, grapes, kiwi fruit, papaya, custard apples or watermelons. The best juices are from root vegetables like carrots, beetroot, celery and celery tops. Follow this diet for 7–21 days and drink plenty of hot water.

- For the *colon* eat soft pears, plums, papaya (with seeds), onion soup, apples (with seeds).
- For the *kidneys and heart* eat watermelons or grapes.
- For the *liver* eat grilled oranges or ripe pineapple.
- For the *stomach* eat apples (without seeds).
- For *all organs* eat peaches, apricots (including the kernel) and nectarines (but only ripe ones).
- To *strengthen* the body eat mangoes, papaya and grapes.

Caution
Apricot kernels in large amounts can be poisonous.

❋ Non-vegetarian cleansing diet for non-allergic people

This simple but delicious diet will improve your sensibility to quality food – provided you follow the guidelines below:

- Take your meals regularly and avoid hurrying.
- Aim to take frequent small meals (large meals are always bad).
- Avoid taking meals when you are tired or cold (lie down, rest and get warm first).
- Eat and chew thoroughly.
- Do not read or do anything else while eating (it interferes with the digestive process).

- Do not use tinned or preserved food, use only fresh items.
- Use garlic, ginger, red onions and seasonings to make the food more tasty.
- Ensure all food is fresh and, if possible, organic (including meat).

You can eat or drink any of the following:

DAIRY PRODUCTS
Milk (prepared in any way – custard, well-cooked milk puddings, milky soups), plain cream, cream soups, butter, eggs (lightly cooked), yoghurt.

FISH AND MEAT
Boiled, steamed or baked, but not fried. Chicken or game should be well cooked, but not fried.

VEGETABLES
Potatoes (well-cooked or mashed), cauliflower together with its greens, spinach, carrots (well-cooked or sieved), tomatoes (fresh or cooked).

FRUIT
If raw, with skins and seeds and not the pips. If cooked, always sieve.

STARCH
Ryebread, crackers, rice, maize, cassava.

DRINKS
Drink sparingly with meals: weak maté tea, dandelion coffee with milk, freshly prepared fruit juices, and a small quantity of light wine with dinner or supper. Avoid cheap wines. Take plenty of water between meals

SOUPS AND MEAT DISHES
Avoid meat soups and rich gravies, twice-cooked meat (leftovers), made-up dishes, pork and all tough meat.

FISH
Avoid salmon, sardines, dried fish.

CONDIMENTS
Use spices, pepper, vinegar, relishes, pickles, sauces and biochemical salt. Learn how to use Indian and Chinese herbs and spices.

Menu suggestions

EVERY DAY: MID-MORNING
Tea or coffee, 1 crispbread with butter.
Tea or coffee, whenever mentioned, should be taken without milk and sugar.

SUNDAY
Breakfast: Scrambled eggs; 1 cracker with butter; tea or coffee.
Lunch: Tomato soup; roast joint, cauliflower or chicory, parsnips; baked pineapple pudding or fresh fruit.
Dinner: Baked fish (halibut or herring), lettuce and leek salad; blue cheese, butter, 1 crispbread; tea or coffee.

MONDAY
Breakfast: Grilled bacon and tomato, 1 cracker with butter; tea or coffee.
Lunch: Melon; grilled (rare) steak, green salad; pears baked in cider, cream.
Dinner: Lamb chop, tomatoes and green vegetables, 1 medium-sized potato, cream cheese, roasted almonds, 1 crispbread or cracker; tea or coffee.

TUESDAY
Breakfast: Poached haddock, 1 crispbread with butter; tea or coffee.
Lunch: White vegetable soup; baked liver and bacon, carrots, green vegetables.
Dinner: Grapefruit or orange; baked gammon or lamb kebabs, parsley, spinach; peaches; tea or coffee.

WEDNESDAY
Breakfast: Boiled egg, 1 cracker or crispbread with butter; tea or coffee.
Lunch: Stuffed tomatoes, cheese salad; baked oranges.
Dinner: Fruit juice; curried lamb stew, chutney, 1 tablespoon boiled white or brown rice, tomato and onion salad; fresh fruit; tea or coffee.

THURSDAY
Breakfast: Grilled kipper, 1 crispbread with butter; tea or coffee.
Lunch: Grapefruit; minced lamb or mutton, green vegetables; cream cheese with celery sticks, 1 crispbread with butter.

Dinner: Bone-marrow broth; Scotch eggs or cold meat, salad; tea or coffee.

FRIDAY

Breakfast: Grilled sausages or bacon, 1 crispbread with butter; tea or coffee.

Lunch: Egg mayonnaise; baked haddock, peas or green beans, tomatoes; fresh fruit.

Dinner: Watercress and mustard soup; omelette with meat or mushrooms, or mutton hotpot, 1 small potato; carob sweet; tea or coffee.

SATURDAY

Breakfast: Gammon or mushrooms, 1 crispbread with butter; tea or coffee.

Lunch: Tomato juice; fried sweetbreads, onions, green vegetables; baked apple and cream.

Dinner: Pear and lettuce salad; lamb chop, green vegetables, peppers; nut cream and honey; tea or coffee.

❋ Drastic slimming plan for rich people

A wealthy patient came to me because he had heard that I prescribed diets as part of my treatments. It was the first occasion that he had consulted a natural healer. He was a generously proportioned man committed to eating meat and drinking alcohol, and it was evident that he needed to lose weight.

Somewhat dramatically, after my examination and diagnosis I gave my patient an envelope. I told him to give it, sealed, to his wife. He received quite a surprise when he was served with steak, champagne and onions 3 times a day.

The instructions inside the envelope were as follows:

- 250g steak
- 450g boiled onions   3 times a day – nothing else.
- ½ bottle of champagne

He was allowed no other liquids apart from the water in which the onions were boiled. By following this slimming plan for 14–21 days, he was able to lose fat and weight without any consequent loss of energy.

❊ Seven-day spring-cleaning diet

As the name suggests, this is a springtime diet. In the same way that we spring-clean our homes after the winter, you can detoxify and cleanse your body from the effects of winter foods, which are often preserved and rich in starch and proteins. To initiate this change of diet, eat only raw food for 1 day before starting the diet.

DAY 1
Fruit juice diluted with distilled or de-calcified water, alternating with clear vegetable soup from seasonally available vegetables. Use 6 cups of diced or grated vegetables for the vegetable soup. Boil with 4 litres of water until 2 litres are left. Drink 1 cup every 2 hours during the day.

DAY 2
As Day 1.

DAY 3
Three meals of fresh fruit only – pineapples, peaches, apples, oranges, grapefruit, pears, etc. Eat mixed fresh fruit if you wish.

DAY 4
As Day 3, plus a glass of instant biological vegetable bouillon at each meal.

DAY 5
Breakfast: fresh fruit and bioyoghurt.
Lunch: large salad comprising lettuce, watercress and grated carrots; raisins and soaked prunes or figs.
Dinner: steamed cabbage and carrots with 50g of marinated tofu – cooked or raw.

DAY 6
Breakfast: fresh fruit with wheatgerm and bioyoghurt.
Lunch: large mixed salad with 3 crispbreads and butter.
Dinner: steamed sprouts or greens, organically grown potatoes baked in their jackets; baked apples stuffed with raisins and cloves.

DAY 7
Design your meal with wholemeal bread, honey, wholewheat cereals, fresh fruit, mixed green salads, fruit juices diluted with water.

Assignment

Take a hot bath every night with 500g Epsom salts (magnesium sulphate), 500g sea salt and 125g bicarbonate of soda. You may also add 1 teaspoon each of mustard powder and paprika. Be careful not to touch or rub your eyes. Stand up slowly to avoid dizziness, then take a cold shower and rub yourself dry with a rough towel. Go straight to bed with warm night clothes.

If a bath is not available, take hot and cold showers. Let the water run on the spine: 3 minutes hot and 1 minute cold. Repeat this cycle 3 times, finishing with a cold shower.

CHAPTER 2

The Circulatory/Lymphatic System

The *circulatory system* deals with distribution. The heart pumps oxygen and nutrients to the body cells via the blood and blood vessels. The blood vessels also transport carbon dioxide (CO_2) and waste products from the cells. Body temperature and the acid/alkaline balance of the body is regulated by the blood. The blood is also able to protect the body by its ability to thicken and clot in an emergency.

The *lymphathic system* has a separate system of pathways that run throughout the entire body. The spleen, thymus, appendix, tonsils and lymph nodes are linked by this system. These organs filter the blood, keeping it clear of bacteria, fungus and viruses, and ensure the cleansing of white blood cells in the spleen. Proteins are returned to the cardiovascular system via the lymphatic system.

Detoxification

Detoxification takes place in the liver. One of the best ways to stimulate a liver detox is to follow a diet of grilled oranges, which are antifungal, antibacterial and antiviral, and contain large amounts of vitamins C and P. When both these vitamins are combined they form a new vitamin called bioflavanoid complex, which has a positive powerful impact on the immune system. When you grill or bake an orange, the pith becomes very mushy and mingles with the flesh; this pap is the most potent part. Cut the oranges in half and place them on the grill with the insides facing the heat. Grill until the flesh starts to turn brown, as if cinnamon had been sprinkled on it.

In addition to its detoxifying effect, this diet is also beneficial for shingles and the treatment of hepatitis A, B and C.

When the liver is unable to detoxify the system effectively, disease can be expressed as herpes, HIV, hepatitis or non-specific urethritis (NSU) – various forms of expression of a partial breakdown in the immune system.

Many people carry the TB virus without suffering from tuberculosis. This could be proven relatively easily by testing the saliva of a cross-section of the population. Conversely, there is a reasonable possibility that a number of people in hospital tuberculosis wards are not TB virus carriers. Confusingly, and controversially, the presence of a virus is not synonymous with the expression of disease – HIV, for example, does not lead to immediate death and is therefore unlikely to be the sole cause of Aids, although in the end most HIV carriers are likely to succumb to it.

Diagnosis of the virus does not always result in the medical prognosis based on that diagnosis, regardless of the faith that we place in the diagnosis/prognosis paradigm favoured by our medical establishment.

❈ Blood-purifying diet

For the first 7 days grill 16 oranges a day. Drink plenty of hot water while eating the oranges. For a further 14 days grill 4 oranges a day at breakfast time. Eat plenty of raw foods during the day. You may also drink nettle tea. Do not mix fruits with vegetables.

Then for 90 days eat grilled oranges for breakfast. At other meals eat 70 per cent of your food raw and 30 per cent cooked. Do not eat any red meat, sugar or wheat, or drink any milk. Drink 4 cups of dandelion coffee and 2 cups of nettle tea a day. Eat plenty of plums, kiwi fruit, red onions, cos (Romaine) lettuce and broccoli – when in season.

Assignments

1 Ensure you get plenty of relaxation and sleep, and take easy walks.
2 Give yourself a few drops of TLC (tender loving care) 4 times a day.
3 Try a dry (friction) bath in the morning and a hot Epsom salts bath (500g) at night. Dead Sea salt baths are also effective.

CHAPTER 3

The Digestive System

The *digestive system* comprises the gastro-intestinal tract (oesophagus, stomach, duodenum, jejunum, ileum), the salivary glands, liver, gall bladder and pancreas. The large colon is part of the excretory system. The function of the digestive system is the mechanical and chemical break-down of foods, which are then transported via the blood to the cells.

Candidiasis or yeast infection is caused by the fungus *candida albicans*, which is present in small amounts in the intestine, genital tract, mouth and throat of a healthy body. When the volume of fungus increas-es, due to an encouraging environment, candidiasis breaks out. Because the fungus travels easily through the bloodstream, illness can occur in many parts of the body. Symptoms include:

- diarrhoea
- colitis and abdominal pain
- constipation
- cancer sores
- muscle and joint pains
- sore throat
- congestion
- dry cough
- numb hands, legs or face
- acne
- vaginitis
- kidney and bladder infections
- arthritis
- depression
- hyperactivity
- hyperthyroidism

One of the most frequent forms of candidiasis is commonly known as thrush – a vaginal infection, accompanied by intense itching and a white cheese-like discharge. Candidiasis can also infect the mouth and throat, resulting in white sores on the tongue, gums and cheeks.

The body is a benign host to the candida fungus. It can be likened to a palace with central heating, abundant nourishment and a welcome sign. A clean-out of the bowels is one of the most effective ways to combat this irritating ailment.

It will pay you dividends to learn more about the process of ingestion, digestion, assimilation and elimination. In breathing, for example, most people use only a third of their lungs' capacity, thus seriously hampering oxygenation. The first lesson is to learn how to exhale air properly: a process over which you have direct and personal control. According to the Chinese energy-meridian philosophy, the colon is connected to the lungs, and because of this connection, albeit indirectly, when you improve your exhalation you will find that almost miraculously the colon begins to empty itself more readily.

I have always maintained that around 70 per cent of the population in Britain above the age of 60–65 are constipated. Certainly, many people of this age take laxatives. Taking laxatives and evacuating the bowels three times a week is regarded by many people as 'normal.' In fact, healthy people have a bowel movement once or twice a day.

The process of evacuation is as follows. Initially urine is passed from the bladder, followed by stools from the bowel. The bowels then release pressure on the bladder, allowing water to be passed a second time – a good sign that the bowels have been emptied properly. If they have not been, the bacteria that remain in the colon are given an opportunity to ferment. Because most of the liquid that we ingest is absorbed by the body through the colon and not via the kidneys, auto-intoxication is the unfortunate result.

An effective means to combat these unfriendly colonic bacteria is to stimulate *acidophilus* bacteria by eating bioyoghurt with rotten bananas. Also caprilic acid (found in coconuts) is known to be a powerful anti yeast/fungal agent. It is available in capsule form, but a cheaper alternative is to grate a coconut to produce coconut milk and drink this on an empty stomach. If the bacteria are causing ulceration, use cabbage and potato juice mixed together. Again, take the mixture when your stomach is empty. Remember, however, that for these treatments to be effective, it is important to first of all empty the lower bowels, where the fermentation is taking place.

Discover for yourself which foods you have allergic reactions to. This will tell you which foods stimulate fermentation in your colon. It could be yeast, sugar, junk food or whatever. You need to find this out for yourself. So stop feeding the bacteria and clean them out of your system.

✳ Banana diet for candida

For 7 days eat 2 rotten overripe black bananas (mashed and with a pinch of pepper) with 250g of bioyoghurt every 2 hours, *or* eat 4 rotten overripe bananas (mashed and with a pinch of pepper) with 500g of bioyoghurt every 4 hours. Remember to drink plenty of hot water.

For breakfast on the next 21 days eat 2 rotten overripe mashed bananas with 250g bioyoghurt and some added pepper. Eat nothing else for 2 hours afterwards. Eat only cooked vegetables during the day. Drink hot water and herb tea. Avoid other drinks, especially stimulants such as coffee, tea, Coca Cola.

For the next 2 months eat 2 rotten bananas with 250g of bioyoghurt (with a pinch of pepper) for breakfast. Wait for 2 hours before eating any other food. For all other meals eat 70 per cent cooked food and 30 per cent raw.

During the whole 3 months avoid the following:

- milk, sugar, wheat and red meat
- yeast in any shape or form – fermented products such as beer, alcohol and cheese and yeast spreads like Marmite (some vitamin supplements, particularly vitamin B, contain brewer's yeast)

Assignments

1　After the first 7 days eat 1 papaya a day and chew 20 black papaya seeds.
2　Take 2 capsules of caprilic acid a day.
3　Drink at least 3 cups of coconut milk a week.
4　Eat more garlic, leeks, red onions, cos (Romaine) lettuce, chives, celery tops and turnip tops.
5　Learn how to breathe out properly. Massage your abdomen when sitting on the toilet.
6　Have a reflexology foot massage to stimulate the lungs and colon.

7 Be tickled for 5 minutes, increasing to 10 a day. Buy funny videos and play them for half an hour a day at least 3 times a week.
8 Dance naked to fast music in front of a mirror for 10 minutes, then laugh until your stomach hurts.

❄ Elimination diet 1

For the first 2 days eat only grapes, with pips and skin. The cheapest white grapes are the best for this purpose. Eat as many as you like. If thirsty, drink water. Practise deep breathing for 10 minutes every day. The 2 days of grapes should be followed by 4 days on the following diet:

ON RISING
The juice of 2 oranges undiluted and unsweetened. Sipped slowly.

BREAKFAST
150–200g grapes or a ripe pear.

MID-MORNING
2 firm but not overripe tomatoes. Eat slowly and chew well.

LUNCH
Small salad, finely chopped lettuce and/or watercress, grated raw carrot, cucumber, chopped onion, chives, mint and parsley. Lemon juice as a dressing if desired. Eat slowly and chew well.

AFTERNOON
Juice of 2 oranges, sipped slowly, or 150g of grapes.

EVENING MEAL
2–3 tomatoes eaten alone and slowly, or a small salad as at midday.

BEFORE RETIRING
Grapes and a ripe pear or peach.

After 4 days on this diet, eat buttered rye-crackers at midday with the salad. The next day eat grated cheese as well as rye-crackers. In the evening eat a small meal of cooked green and root vegetables with scrambled egg. Thereafter you can begin to progress to a full diet. Meals must be kept small and be well masticated. The main basis of meals should be fruit and salad, eggs, white fish, cheese and nuts, with lean white meat occasionally. Breakfast should always consist of fresh fruit. For dessert have a few dried dates or figs or 1 teaspoon of maple syrup. Your evening meal should be prepared with steamed root vegetables.

Assignments

1 Ensure that you empty your bowels every day.
2 Each day rub down your spine with a cold sponge followed by brisk drying with a rough towel.
3 Take a hot bath every night with 500g Epsom salts (magnesium sulphate). Stay in the bath for 20–30 minutes. Have the water as hot as you can bear it. Stay in the bath while you drain the water. Get up slowly and then take a cold shower – over your entire body. Rub yourself dry with a rough towel. Put on warm clothing and rest for at least 1 hour.

❋ Elimination diet 2

BREAKFAST
Any fresh fruit such as grapefruit, oranges, grapes and, occasionally, grated apples. A few nuts and raisins or dates. If fruit disagrees with you at any time by producing acid, bake the fruit. You might well find that you begin to suffer from excessive bloating as a reaction to the fruit. In this instance either bake the fruit or eliminate it from your diet.

LUNCH
Any salad in season – such as lettuce, cress, grated carrot, beetroot, cucumber and raw marrow – with toast, wholemeal biscuits, milled nuts, dried fruits, prunes, figs, dates, raisins and honey. Occasionally slippery elm, honey, cream and sultanas may be added. Check that there is no wheat in the ingredients that you purchase.

EVENING MEAL
Cooked vegetables followed by baked fruit.

Eat all meals dry – only drink between meals.

❋ 'Dry' elimination diet

A dry fast will quite fiercely expel fluids from the body. It is not easy to sustain as it results in a degree of suffering, including a dry tongue, though I often regard such suffering as a necessary wake-up call to the system. A dry fast will provide the body with rest, which is especially useful when the liver is in bad shape.

If the body retains stagnant water, this indicates that it is either too alkaline or too acidic. A dry fast will rapidly determine your body orientation, alkaline or acidic, through taste and smell. It is an effective cure for people with excess fluid in the body. This condition is usually indicated by puffiness in the arms, hands and feet. Because the kidneys control the joints, water is mostly retained in the thighs, ankles, knees, elbows, wrists and shoulders. Swollen joints are an indication that they are retaining toxins. Water retention results in skin colouration – red, yellow or blue. There is no colouration if the distention is caused by fat rather than water retention. If there is accompanying pain, the water is diluting the toxins. It is more useful to discover the reason for this than to just treat the symptom.

I recommend the following diet for 7–10 days.

8.00 Three slices dry wholemeal toast (preferably stale bread, 3–4 days old).

13.00 Same as above.

19.00 A couple of wholemeal biscuits. Do not drink until about 21.00 when you can have a glass (500ml) of organic cider.

Assignments

1 Take hot and cold showers on the spine and long brisk walks.
2 Have a foot massage to stimulate the lungs and colon.
3 Have an enema every alternate day using 2 litres of warm water and 50ml of olive oil.

❈ Seven-day elimination diet

This diet consists of a broth that should be produced daily, made up from fresh vegetables, high in alkalinity and rich in vitamins. If possible the diet should be accompanied by 2 or 3 glasses of freshly juiced vegetables. Non-starchy fresh fruit such as apples, pears, peaches, oranges, grapefruit and pineapples are also beneficial, as are herbal teas such as peppermint, strawberry and raspberry.

Make the broth by putting the following into 500ml of cold water:

- 500g celery (3 cups when finely shredded)
- 500g carrots (3 cups when finely shredded)
- 500g raw beetroot with green tops (3 cups when finely shredded)
- 125g spinach (1 cup when finely shredded)
- 25g parsley (¼ cup when finely shredded)
- biochemical salt
- Marmite or organic vegetable stock to taste

The cooking time is crucial in the preparation of this broth. Bring the vegetables to the boil slowly over a 20-minute period. After the boiling point has been reached, allow the broth to simmer for 5–10 minutes (5 minutes is sufficient for finely shredded vegetables). The potency of the broth can be increased by adding more finely chopped raw vegetables or herbs.

ON RISING
Drink a glass of one of the following juices: grapefruit, orange, pineapple, unsweetened apple, tomato, any fresh vegetable. If you usually fail to achieve an effective bowel movement, prepare a mixture of watermelon and raw beetroot juice and drink first thing in the morning.

11.00
A bowl of broth warmed up – season by adding biochemical salt, paprika and nutmeg powder.

LUNCH
A large cup of broth, fresh fruit or vegetable salad and, if still hungry, a dessert of fresh or stewed fruit.

16.00
A large glass of fresh fruit juice or vegetable juice followed by a bowl of broth about half an hour later.

DINNER
Broth followed by a large salad, dessert of fresh or stewed fruit or a baked apple.

BEFORE RETIRING
A herbal laxative should be taken each night. To a cup of warm water add:

- 1 teaspoon slippery elm
- 1 teaspoon fenugreek powder
- 1 teaspoon psyllium husks

Assignments

1 Learn to breathe fully. Use the abdomen to breathe in and out, expelling completely all the air in the lungs. Do not pause between breaths.
2 Take long walks.
3 Take hot and cold showers, letting the water run onto the spine.
4 Have a foot massage to stimulate colon and lungs.

❋ Diet for gall bladder and gallstones

The gall bladder contains bile, a dense liquid consisting principally of cholesterol, bile salts and lecithin. Bile is the substance that breaks down fats in the body; it is produced in the liver. Appetisers are foods and drinks that stimulate the gall bladder to release sufficient bile to digest fatty meals. An inability to do this results in indigestion. Over-production of bile causes diarrhoea, whereas under-production causes constipation. This diet is recommended for the stimulation of the gall bladder. It will also have a beneficial effect on its overall performance.

ON RISING
Glass of hot water.

8.00   1 grilled grapefruit or 2 grilled oranges or a cup of stewed prunes.

10.30   Cup of soya milk with 1 teaspoon of Marmite.

12.00   Glass of still mineral water.

13.00 White fish (grilled or steamed), green salad with 1 dessertspoon olive oil, 1 or 2 slices of wholemeal bread; stewed or raw fruit.

16.00 One cup of green China tea.

18.00 Glass of mineral water.

19.15 12 garlic-soaked olives 15 minutes before the evening meal.

19.30 Clear soup (no fat); grilled cutlet or chicken, small portion of mashed potato with skin, green vegetable with 1 teaspoon of olive oil; stewed or raw fruit; glass of hot water with slice of lemon or cup of dandelion (leaf or root) tea.

Follow this diet for 3 weeks.

Gallstones

Gallstones are crystallized bile. The lemon/olive oil treatment will stimulate the gall bladder to release it. It can be most painful if the gallstone enters the intestinal tract. Should this happen, drink some slippery elm to smooth its path.

For the 6 days of this diet follow this regimen first thing in the morning:

Day 1:   Drink the juice of 2 lemons.
Day 2:   Drink the juice of 4 lemons.
Days 3–5: Increase the number of lemons by 2 each day.
Day 6:   Drink the juice of 6 lemons and an equal amount of cold-pressed olive oil *in the evening* before going to bed. Then drink a cup of hot water with 1 tablespoon of Epsom salts. The stones should pass out of the body in either vomit or stools.

Assignments

1 Practise expressing your feelings by getting angry and pulling faces in front of the mirror for 10 minutes each day. (Gall bladder problems are connected with anger in that angry people tend to produce more bile.)
2 Take a cold sitz bath for 3 minutes before bed.
3 Have a foot massage to stimulate kidney, bladder, liver and gall bladder.
4 Take a coffee enema to cleanse the colon.

❋ Diet for duodenal/gastric ulcers and chronic intestinal inflammation

Hydrochloric acid (HCl) is a beneficial substance which kills off many harmful bacteria that enter the stomach in food. In Eastern philosophy, the stomach is connected to the spleen by energy meridians. Both organs are also affected by apprehension, worry and anxiety. Spleen energy is therefore seen to have an influence on the production of HCl, an excess of which will burn the stomach walls and the duodenum. The symptoms are wind and problems with digestion.

You will need 16 rotten overripe bananas daily. Every 2 hours throughout the day alternate between 2 bananas mashed together with 125g of bioyoghurt and 4 bananas mashed together with 250g of bioyoghurt. Drink plenty of hot water.

AFTER 14 DAYS
Breakfast: Banana and bioyoghurt.
Lunch: Raw food with slippery elm food drink.
Dinner: Cooked and puréed vegetables.

Assignments

1 Drink 6 cups of cos (Romaine) lettuce soup with nutmeg powder. (1 lettuce, chopped fine, added to 12 cups of water, boils down to 6 cups.)
2 Take hot and cold showers on the spine.
3 Sing for 10 minutes in the morning and in the evening.
4 Be tickled for 3 minutes twice a day.

Duodenal ulcers

The following diet is recommended if you have been diagnosed as having a duodenal ulcer.

Take soups made with milk and strained vegetables or soft green vegetables, preferably steamed. Eat slippery elm malted food 3 times a day. Drink biological instant bouillon and/or cos (Romaine) lettuce soup. Bread should be eaten sparingly and only in the form of oven toast, very dry and crisp.

Avoid raw fruits and vegetables. All alcoholic drinks and smoking are strictly forbidden.

Drink the following on an empty stomach:

- 25ml raw potato juice – do not skin the potatoes
- 25ml raw green cabbage juice

Prepare this juice fresh with a vegetable juicer and *not* in a blender.

Assignments

1 Take 2 large sticks and conduct music with a fast rhythm for 10 minutes in the morning and 10 minutes in the evening.
2 Take a cold sitz bath 3 minutes before bed.
3 Laugh till your stomach hurts.

✤ Diet for intestinal ulcers

FOR 7 DAYS: 16–20 overripe bananas, nothing else.

FOR 7 DAYS: every 2 hours, 2 bananas with 100g bioyoghurt mashed, or every 4 hours, 4 bananas with 200g bioyoghurt mashed. Drink camomile tea and 8–12 cups of hot water.

FOR 14 DAYS: 4 overripe bananas with 200g yoghurt for breakfast. Eat only fruits – mixed – and no vegetables throughout the day. Drink 8–12 cups of hot water.

FOR 14 DAYS: 4 rotten bananas with 200g yoghurt for breakfast. Eat raw foods only. Do not mix fruits with vegetables.

FOR 90 DAYS: 4 rotten bananas with 200g yoghurt for breakfast. Eat 70 per cent raw food and 30 per cent cooked. Drink hot water with a slice of lemon or spoon of molasses.

CHAPTER 4

The Endocrine System

The two systems responsible for the co-ordination of processes in the body are the nervous system and the endocrine system. While the nervous system acts fast and precisely, the endocrine system acts more slowly. The hormones which act as the messengers of the endocrine system are produced in various glands – the pineal, pituitary, parathyroids, thyroid, thymus, adrenals, Islets of Langerhans, pancreas, ovaries and testes. These glands regulate body action by secreting hormones via the circulatory system – the blood and blood vessels – to the target organs.

The *pineal gland* is regulated by sunlight and geomagnetic fields. It is important for the integration of body cycles (menstruation, sleep and waking rhythm). It controls the metabolism, behaviour and physiological functions and influences ageing and chronic diseases.

The *hypophysis* connects the nervous system and the endocrine system. It modulates the activity of the pituitary glands. It produces hormones to release (-liberin) hormones, and hormones to inhibit further production (-statin) of hormones. The hypophysis also produces oxytocin and an antidiuretic hormone. The former influences the production of mother's milk while the latter holds back water in the kidneys. For further information refer to the *Merck Manual*, p. 985.

The thyroid

Iodine is required for the production of the thyroid hormones (thyroxine and tri-iodothyronine). Nutrients which are high in iodine are iodized salts, water, seafood, salt-water fish and kelp; also, arame, algae and seaweed. In smaller amounts it is found in asparagus, pulses, garlic, lima beans, mushrooms, sesame seeds and soya beans. Foods that block the intake of iodine are Brussels sprouts, cabbage, cauliflower, peaches, pears, spinach, kale and turnips. In the case of cretinism (lack of thyroxine), these foods should only be eaten in small amounts.

❊ Diet for hyperthyroidism

Menu suggestions

SUNDAY

Breakfast: 1 orange with a few dates or dried figs, baked apple(s) and a cup of organic vegetable bouillon.

Lunch: Small salad of lettuce, tomato, radishes and cress with some thin slices of lean lamb or veal or chicken, 2 potatoes boiled in their skins, carrots; fresh fruit.

Dinner: Vegetable purée with a few slices of wholemeal bread with 12g of butter.

MONDAY

Breakfast: Grapefruit with a cup of mint tea and 1 sheet of nori.

Lunch: Steamed cod or turbot with parsley and wholemeal bread and butter.

Dinner: Fresh green salad with an apple or pear; 1 cup of organic vegetable bouillon.

TUESDAY

Breakfast: Soaked prunes or figs.

Lunch: Small lamb cutlet with steamed spinach and celery; fresh fruit with a little thin cream.

Dinner: Raw mixed salad with wholemeal bread and 12g butter and a cup of organic vegetable bouillon.

WEDNESDAY

Breakfast: 1 orange or 3 kiwi fruit with a cup of mint tea and 1 sheet of nori.

Lunch: Steamed white fish with baked cauliflower, carrots and a boiled potato (eat the skin as well); a baked apple.

Dinner: Raw mixed salad with dressing of pure honey, olive oil and lemon juice; an apple or a pear.

THURSDAY

Breakfast: 2 thin rashers of grilled bacon and a grilled tomato; mint tea.

Lunch: Small lamb cutlet or small portion of veal or chicken with steamed greens and carrots; a baked apple.

Dinner: Steamed spinach with wholemeal bread and 12g butter and a cup of vegetable bouillon.

FRIDAY

Breakfast: Fresh fruit salad with bioyoghurt; dandelion coffee; 1 sheet of nori.

Lunch: Steamed white fish, a boiled potato (with its skin) and one steamed green vegetable; an apple, pear or orange.

Dinner: Purée of vegetables with spinach; wholemeal bread and butter and Marmite or Vecon.

SATURDAY

Breakfast: Fresh fruit (only one kind of fruit at a time) and a cup of organic vegetable bouillon.

Lunch: Steamed fish or stewed hotpot with steamed green vegetables; a pear or apple.

Dinner: Large green salad; boiled cauliflower with sesame sauce; a cup of organic vegetable bouillon.

CHAPTER 5

The Functional System

❋ Eye improvement diet

Vitamin A is required to improve the eyesight. The best sources of vitamin A are fish liver oils, parsley, escarole (endive family), egg yolks, calves' liver, carrots, cream cheese, spinach and turnip greens. The next best sources are: butter, biocheese, radish tops, cream, apricots, prunes, kale, beet greens, beetroot, broccoli and sweet peppers (red, yellow, green).

Vitamin B also contributes to the wellbeing of the eyes. The best sources of vitamin B are brewer's yeast, milk, eggs, beet greens, turnip greens, soya beans and broccoli. The next best sources are spinach, lettuce, cabbage, kidneys, beef, veal and liver.

Menu suggestions

BREAKFAST
Stewed fruit; dandelion coffee; wholemeal cereal or cream.

LUNCH
Raw carrot salad, omelette, wholemeal bread with butter or margarine; fresh fruit drinks or dandelion coffee, if desired.

DINNER
Vegetable juice; grilled organic calves' liver, onions, carrots, potatoes in jackets; prunes or apricots.

Exercises to strengthen the eyes

Sit in a straight-backed chair or in an upright position in bed. Relax, and without moving your body or shoulders:

1 Move your head in a complete circle 7 times clockwise and 7 times anti-clockwise.
2 Move your head from left to right 7 times.
3 Move your head up and down 7 times.
4 Move your eyes in a circular motion without moving the head 7 times, then reverse, 7 times, first clockwise and then anti-clockwise.
5 Look up 7 times.
6 Look down 7 times.
7 Look from upper right to lower left 7 times.
8 Look from upper left to lower right 7 times.
9 Shut your eyes as tightly as possible and then open them as wide as you can 7 times.
10 Pin a small written statement on a wall. Walk backwards and read it until the writing becomes blurred. Walk toward the statement until your nose almost touches the wall and you can still see the statement.
11 Read *Natural Vision Improvement* by Janet Goodrich.

Assignments

1 Have hot and cold showers over the spine.
2 Eat raw liver (150g 3 times week) from an organic butcher. Eat more barley, soya beans, mackerel and oysters.
3 Fall in love with yourself, and meditate on the third eye – between the eyebrows on the forehead.
4 Read the above book – it may be possible to learn to see without spectacles.
5 Try Alexander technique lessons to correct your body posture.
6 Wash your eyes with your midstream urine before bed.
7 Drink 250ml freshly pressed carrot juice in the morning and evening.
8 Take vitamins A and D (10,000 units).
9 Practise shadow boxing while making a 'psshh' sound by pursing the lips for 10 minutes to the rhythm of fast and lively music. Force the air out of your lungs with each punch.

CHAPTER 6

The Immune System

It is generally inadvisable to eat food containing mutated gluten. But in order to render starch or grain free of gluten, it is necessary to remove the gluten chemically. Most processed foods are not healthy and it is best to avoid them. Margarine is therefore less healthy than butter; instant coffee is less healthy than ground coffee; and in my opinion and that of other holistic practitioners, cooking in the microwave is less healthy than frying and other more conventional cooking methods. The price for the convenience of the microwave is food that is deprived of nutrition. Food cooked in this way can also lead to the development of allergies.

Allergies

Many people suffer from allergies as a result of consuming gluten. More and more people are affected as a result of 40 years of meddling with the soil and using artificial fertilisers. It has given gluten the opportunity to mutate. If wheat and other grains were grown organically, the problem of gluten-allergies would be minimized and possibly vanish completely.

An allergy is a sign that the body is producing toxins in reaction to certain substances. You can usually detect a gluten allergy by the following symptoms:

- irritated nasal passages
- vaginal irritation
- diarrhoea

- indigestion with bloating
- bitter taste in the mouth
- scratching
- itching
- sore eyes
- sneezing
- constant catarrh
- sugar imbalance

These symptoms are a sign that the body is becoming unable to cope with processed food and the accumulation of toxins. You will be healthier if you can remove the gluten-related toxins from the body. It would, however, be helpful to cleanse the body beforehand with an elimination diet.

A colon and liver detox is the most effective way to rid the body of these toxins. One of the best ways to assist these organs is by using the lungs to breathe more efficiently. According to the Chinese five-element cycle, the three relevant elements here are *metal* (colon and lungs), *wood* (the liver) and *water* (the kidneys). When the colon and lungs are not functioning effectively, the metal (colon and lungs) gradually destroys the wood (the liver). Improper functioning of the colon and liver increases the toxicity of the body, resulting in the liver, the only organ that purifies the blood, becoming exhausted. Lungs and colon are the mother of the kidneys and are intended to nourish them. An insufficient amount of energy to perform this operation will result in the kidneys functioning deficiently. This can result in dehydration of the body, impurity of the blood from insufficient cleansing, a lack of minerals, high blood pressure and back ache. So, help yourself by learning to breathe out more effectively.

First, eliminate carbon dioxide and carbon monoxide from the lungs. Whilst performing regular breathing exercises, undergo an elimination diet (7-Day Spring-cleaning Diet, Elimination Diet 1 or 2, Grape Diet, or Grape and Fruit Diet) to cleanse the colon. When the colon is empty and clean, the liver will once again properly purify the system. After this cleansing you can begin to change your diet by omitting foods which contain gluten.

❋ Gluten-free diet

Gluten is the protein present in wheat and rye. These two cereals, and products made from them, should be avoided (ie, wheat flour, crackers, cakes, pasta, biscuits, semolina, puffed wheat, barley and oats). The best foods to eat are millet, wild rice, yellow corn and buckwheat. You may also eat cornflakes, rice, cornflour, sago, rice crispies, custard powder, tapioca and arrowroot.

Gluten-free bread and biscuits are available at most health food stores.

The following foods should be eaten daily in adequate amounts to provide a balanced diet: fresh meats, fish, cheese, eggs, fresh fruit and vegetables, butter, tofu and sprouted grain seeds.

Whenever possible, use sunflower or safflower seed oil for salads and cooking. When frying, use oil only once and then throw it away. Once cooked, oil will oxidize.

CHAPTER 7

The Metabolic System

❊ Alkaline diet for arthritis and degenerative diseases

Alkalinity and acidity

In terms of alkalinity and acidity, indicated by the pH factor, distilled water is neutral. The pH norm is 7.0; anything below indicates acidity and higher levels indicate alkalinity. The ideal pH range for saliva and urine is 6.0 to 6.8 which indicates that the body is slightly acidic. A pH factor below 6.0 is considered too acidic, and a pH above 6.8 too alkaline. People suffering from arthritis are too acidic.

Indications of too much acidity are heart-burn, from food that is too acidic, and water retention. Indications of alkalinity are lethargy and water retention – the body's response in order to protect the cells. An excess of alkaline kills off body cells.

If in doubt, have a test performed on your urine and saliva to determine your pH level.

If you suffer from arthritic complaints it is advisable to eat 100 per cent alkaline-forming foods for a period of 3 months. Thereafter balance your food intake with a constant diet of 80 per cent alkaline and 20 per cent acid-forming foods. This advice applies too if you wish to prevent degenerative diseases. Many experiments have shown that people with a predominantly alkaline body are less prone to disease and have a greater self-healing ability.

Although citrus fruits are acidic in taste, they become alkaline when digested and restore the alkaline balance in the body. Citrus fruits contain potassium citrate and they lose their original acidity during oxidation and become alkaline carbohydrates. Citrus fruits such as oranges, grapefruit, lemons and limes also stimulate peptic activity by up to 50 per cent. They assist people who do not produce sufficient gastric juices and who suffer from gastric disorders such as dyspepsia. All of these beneficial qualities can be attributed only to *fresh* citrus fruit. When citrus juice is canned or bottled it becomes acid-forming.

Coffee is acid-producing. Most grains are acid-forming, including buckwheat, barley, wheat, quinoa, corn, oats, rye, rice. The exception is millet.

buy

Acidity or alkalinity is determined by the organic salts a food contains.

Acid-binding organic salts	Acid-forming organic salts
Potassium	Sulphur
Iron	Phosphorus
Sodium	Silicon
Calcium	Chlorine
Magnesium	

Alkaline-forming foods

Almonds
Apples, raw and cooked
Apricots (fresh or tinned)
Artichokes (Jerusalem artichokes become acidic when cooked)

Bananas, raw and cooked
Beans, green and fresh
Beetroot
Berries (raw)
Blackeye beans
Breadfruit
Broccoli

Cabbage
Carob
Carrots
Cassava
Cauliflower florets (the white stem is acid-forming because of its high sulphur content)
Celery
Chives
Cider
Cider vinegar
Coleslaw
Cos (Romaine) lettuce
Cress (garden cress, watercress, mustard)
Cucumbers

Daikon (Japanese radish)
Dandelion, fresh

Endives

Figs, fresh (dried figs are
    acid-forming)

Grapefruit
Guavas

Hazelnuts
Herbs, fresh
Honey
Horseradish

Kale
Kohlrabi
Kumquats

Leeks
Limburger cheese
Loquats

Maple syrup
Melons
Millet
Milk, skimmed
Molasses
Mushrooms
Mustard
Mustard leaves

Okra
Olives
Onions, raw
Oysters

Pears
Peas, fresh
Pickles (when oil and garlic
    and vinegar are used they are
    acid-forming, whereas with
    lemon the pickles are
    alkaline-forming)
Potatoes, with the skin
Pumpkins

Radishes

Sauerkraut
Seaweed (Nori, Kombu, Iziki,
    Wakame, etc)
Spinach, raw (it produces uric acid
    when cooked)
Squash
Swiss cheese

Tamarind
Turnips, with skin and leaves

Watermelons

Yoghurt from skimmed milk

● **RECOMMENDED ALKALIZING GREEN DRINK:**
Take any green food: tops of beets, celery, leeks, turnips, mustard plants,
nettles, cos (Romaine) lettuce. Chop into small pieces or shred and add to
3 litres of water. Boil down to 1½ litres and drink during the day. Keep it
hot in a thermos flask. This drink is very alkalizing; it also provides the
body with chlorophyll and minerals such as zinc, copper and iron which
build up the red blood cells.

❋ Pineapple diet for arthritis and gout

When suffering from acute arthritis or gout, try a pineapple monofast for 7 days. Ensure that the pineapples are very ripe and that the acidic core is removed.

Then eat raw food for at least 1 month and continue to eat pineapple for breakfast.

– Avoid sugar or wheat products.
– Drink plentiful amounts of bottled water.
– Avoid all fizzy drinks as they contain saccharine.

Ensure a plentiful supply of ripe pineapples *before* beginning the diet, remembering to cut out the acidic parts. (When ripe pineapples are unavailable, switch to the potato peel diet described below.) Also take homoeopathic tissue salts as advised by a homoeopath.

RECIPE
Squeeze the juice from:

- 3 pineapples
- 3 oranges
- 3 lemons
- 3 grapefruit

Put the juice in a jar with a lid. Put the pineapple skins with the pips of the oranges, lemons and grapefruit into a blender and pulp. Place in a glass basin and add 450ml of cold water. Leave overnight. The next day mix with the juice and strain. Then pour 250ml of boiling water into an earthenware or china receptacle and add the following ingredients:

- 50g cream of tartar (citric acid)
- 50g Epsom salts (edible)
- 25g bicarbonate of soda

Dissolve this mixture in the water and leave to cool. (As cream of tartar does not mix readily, you will need to stir it in well and shake the mixture vigorously before taking.) Mix with the juice and bottle. Drink a glass (150ml) from time to time each day on an empty stomach for 27 weeks. By that time your body will have thrown off all stiffness in the joints.

As a general rule it is safer to avoid eating oranges and lemons on their own if you suffer from arthritis since they tend to affect the calcium balance of the body.

✳ Diet for rheumatoid spondylitis

Rheumatoid spondylitis is a form of arthritis in which the joints of the spinal column become inflamed. Symptoms vary in intensity while it is in the active or progressive phase, and even when the disease is no longer active the patient is left with bad posture or misalignment of the spinal column.

Together with breathing exercises, postural training, rest and home water treatments, diet is an important part of the natural treatment.

Assignment

Eat 6 portions of raw or cooked vegetables with 2 portions of cooked fruit at mealtimes, and 2 portions of proteins such as beans and lentils, tofu, lean meat or fish occasionally.

Potato peel diet

This diet is particularly suitable for sufferers of rheumatoid spondylitis and rheumatoid arthritis.

Eat 1kg of potato peel a day – about 6kg of potatoes. The peel, which should be about 1cm thick, must be cooked, mashed and eaten as a soup. Eat for 7–14 days, depending on how you feel.

This diet brings to mind a woman who came to my surgery in Suryodaya in a wheelchair with severe arthritic problems. After recommending a 2-week potato peel diet, I was away in India for 6 weeks. Upon my return, I learned to my surprise that the woman had continued the diet beyond the 2 weeks. To my further delight, she came to visit me moving freely and dancing.

If there is an excess of uric acid in the body, the pineapple diet would be more appropriate.

Assignments

1 Drink plenty of water.
2 Sing, dance and laugh to fast music.
3 Learn to cook with more garlic, ginger, red onions and condiments. They are beneficial and, of course, make food tastier.

❃ Treatment for traumatic arthritis (osteoarthritis)

An example of this condition is an inflamed finger. Crush 4 ice cubes and put *directly* on the swollen part: the direct contact of the ice with the skin is an important healing factor. Cover with a cloth. You will experience five different stages: wet, cold, pain, burning, numbness. Remove the ice when the inflamed area feels numb. Rub tea tree oil in a circular motion into the numbed skin.

Drink lots of bottled water. *Do not* drink wine; if you require alcohol, drink only champagne and vodka. Cut out all fizzy drinks as they contain saccharine.

❃ Eating advice for the overweight

Fat is used to keep the body warm and to provide fat cushions. When you accumulate fat, your body starts depositing and storing it. This process can have unpleasant consequences – such as obesity and the risk of heart attacks – especially for people with a high level of cholesterol in the blood.

An overweight person is desperately in need of a low-fat diet. It is healthier for a fat person to eat unsaturated fats and cold-pressed oils than lards or animal-fats. But many people find eating fat satisfying: it provides a full-up feeling. To overcome this, follow these guidelines:

– Eat to satisfy half your hunger.
– Avoid starch (bread, pasta, biscuits, pastries, grains).
– Eat only when you feel hungry, not because it is time to eat.
– Eat sitting down, do nothing else: no reading, telephone calls, talking, etc.
– Eat more pungent, hot, putrid, astringent, bitter foods.
– Cut down on sweet, sour, salty foods.

Assignments

1 Every evening take a very hot bath with 500g Epsom salts and 100g sea salt. Stay in the bath for 30 minutes. Drain the water and have a cold shower. Rub yourself dry and go straight to bed.

2 Take tissue salts – Nat. Mur. 6, 3 tablets under the tongue – before going to bed.

3 Eat 4 grilled oranges for breakfast *every day* for 1 year. Cut them into halves and grill them. Scoop out the contents and leave the skin. The one year duration allows the body to pass through all the seasons.

4 Drink 2–3 litres of fresh undiluted juice during the day, made from equal quantities of the following juices:
- carrot
- celery
- spinach
- cucumber

Add a pinch each of cumin powder, nutmeg powder, salt.

5 Eat raw foods during the day and have a cooked evening meal. Avoid milk, sugar, wheat, red meat. Eat a bunch of radishes with leaves while drinking the juice and concentrate on one thought for 10 minutes a day.

❋ Low-fat/high-protein sports diet

ON WAKING
Place the juice of a whole lemon and the juice of a whole orange in a tumbler of hot water, allow to cool and drink first thing in the morning with 1 tablespoon of fructose. If fruit is not obtainable, use plain water.

BREAKFAST (1)
Choice of ½ grapefruit, orange, apple or stewed prunes; 1 or 2 soft boiled, poached or scrambled eggs; cod, wholemeal bread with butter; cup of tea or dandelion coffee.

or

BREAKFAST (2)
Mixed fruit salad, cut up small, with seedless raisins, covered with ground or ordinary nuts; 25g of sesame seeds; 1 or 2 glasses of fruit juice.

LUNCH
1 or 2 slices of wholemeal bread with fresh butter; tomato and green salad; fruit or fruit salad; glass of fruit juice.

TEA
Cup of tea with buttered rusk or cracker.

DINNER
Pulped cream soup; choice of lean meat, fish, or omelette with potatoes and green salad or mixed vegetable salad; choice of fruit salad or stewed fruit, or pudding made with tapioca, semolina or macaroni.

Avoid all starchy foods, white bread, white sugar, white flour, pickles, vinegar, pastries, sausages; everything that comes out of tins, preserved foods, fried foods, and follow the above-mentioned diet as closely as is convenient. Eat plenty of pomegranates, figs, oranges, ground almonds, cabbage, spinach, carrots, tomatoes, grapes, sesame seeds.

Assignment

Learn how to breathe out properly (see p. 54).

❋ Dietary advice for hyperglycaemia/high blood sugar (diabetes)

Although diabetes can be genetic, it is generally brought on by a shock or a traumatic experience, such as an accident. In the case of infantile diabetes, it will often be discovered that the mother experienced a shock or other problems during pregnancy. In older people diabetes is often the result of an inadequate diet with an excess of starch. Diabetes is caused by the failure of the pancreas to produce insulin. A cure is unlikely to be effective while insulin is being injected because external injections will generally stop the Islets of Langerhans (the insulin-producing gland in the pancreas) from producing the body's own insulin. Unfortunate side-effects of insulin injections are a reduced capacity to deal with infections and varicose ulcers.

A diet that is rich in fats, saturated or unsaturated, is particularly unhealthy for diabetics. Excessive levels of fat in the blood inhibit the body from using and metabolizing sugar and producing ketones. As a result the sugar (glucose) passes out of the body in urine without having been metabolized (used) by the body. For this reason the sugar level will always tend to be high in a nascent diabetic.

As the kidneys note the high sugar level passing through, a message is passed to the pancreas to produce more insulin. The role of insulin is to reduce and regulate the blood sugar level. The insulin converts the glucose (sugar) into glycogen. The resultant glycogen is then stored in the liver as an energy reserve. But the excessive amount of insulin that has been called for causes such a rapid drop in the blood sugar level that the body in desperation calls for more sugar or fatty acid. And so the cycle continues: high sugar level, followed by an excess of insulin production, rapid drop in the blood sugar level and consequently a demand for more sugar and starch – until eventually the body is either unable to produce sufficient insulin or the insulin that it does produce cannot properly regulate the blood sugar level.

Diabetics need to begin treatment by greatly reducing their sugar intake while simultaneously reducing the amount of injected insulin in small graduated steps – but only under medical supervision. Many diabetics, however, prefer to continue eating foods that contain sugar and to continue the injections.

An alternative is to develop other tastes – sweet is just one out of eight tastes (see Appendix A). It is perfectly possible for anybody to develop a taste balance where sugar is no longer predominant.

Colonic irrigation will remove debris and prevent auto-intoxication. It will also remove a false hunger for sugar. The colon has four main sections: the iliocaecal valve, hepatic flexure, splenic flexure and the sigmoid. The splenic flexure is a bend on the left side of the abdomen where blockages often occur. When this happens, the colon dilates and impacts upon the pancreas and spleen, stopping them from working properly. The remedy in the first instance is to clean the system by emptying the transverse colon.

Assignments

1 Have a benefical massage.
2 Eat more bitter and astringent food, which is high in protein and minerals, and reduce your intake of starch and sugar. Sometimes the need for sugar is a pseudo-hunger – a habit.
3 Try homoeopathic remedies.

4 Pay attention to your spleen and stomach – both need love.
5 Eat 6–8 kiwi fruits, including the skin, and no other food for breakfast. Cut the kiwi in half or quarters and add a pinch of salt and black pepper. Do this regularly for 3 months. Kiwi fruit with skin is the only fruit that should be eaten by diabetics seeking a cure. Eating 3–4kg of kiwi fruit a day should bring down the sugar level as they have anti-sugar properties. They increase the secretion of insulin by inducing the Islets of Langerhans to produce more.
6 Learn how to breathe out.
7 Learn how to relax.
8 Understand how diabetes is triggered.

CHAPTER 8

The Neurological System

❊ Blood-pressure-balancing diet

This diet is intended to deal with hypertension and high blood pressure.

BREAKFAST
8 tomatoes or ½ grapefruit or stewed prunes or fruit in season; 1 egg (soft boiled or poached); cup of mint tea or dandelion coffee.

LUNCH
Two vegetables (most fresh vegetables are suitable), raw or cooked; choice of: peas, beans, spinach, cauliflower, asparagus tips, celery, lettuce, turnips, sprouts, potatoes, beetroots, kohlrabi or broccoli; salad.

DINNER
Cream soup or clear vegetable broth; choice of white fish, lamb chops or chicken breast and mutton – fresh lean parts only; 1 potato, 1 green vegetable, 1 portion of wild rice.

TEA
China or Ceylon or maté tea.

Avoid alcoholic beverages, fatty meat and sausages, food that has been cooked twice, all food made with white flour, smoking, aluminium utensils, overeating and eating late at night.

Assignments

1 Take hot and cold showers on the spine. Finish with a cold shower.
2 Practise breathing exercises before bed and upon rising.
3 Learn how to use herbs and spices for cooking.

❋ Diet for brain fatigue and the central nervous system

The central nervous system (CNS) consists of the brain, the spinal chord and spinal fluid, and nerves. Its basic function is to regulate the body functions through nerve impulses. The CNS provides sensory perception and motor response.

This diet will not *cure* any of the following disorders, but it will help to minimize the effect of the symptoms:

- neuralgia – all forms
- sleep disorders
- vertigo
- headaches
- impaired consciousness
- cerebrovascular disease
- meningitis and encephalitis
- brain abscesses
- CNS neoplasms
- tremors
- choleric disorders
- paralysis
- nerve root disorders
- muscular atrophy

BREAKFAST
2 tablespoons of sesame seeds soaked in water overnight *or* 20 pecan nuts soaked overnight *or* 20 almonds soaked overnight and peeled, and ripe raw or dried (soaked overnight) fruit.

MIDDAY
25–50g cream cheese, raw salad (including any palatable raw vegetables, shredded, grated, or minced) with walnut oil and lemon juice dressing. Salads make the gastric juices work. Follow it with 75–100g of dried fruit, preferably apples, dates and pineapples.

EVENING
Wholemeal bread and butter or cereal with cream. Salad again with nuts, cream cheese or honey. Eat half a cup of boiled millet.

NIGHT
Cup of instant vegetable bouillon

DRINKS
Drink about 500–750ml of liquids a day between meals. The following are all acceptable: barley water, dandelion coffee, bran tea or rice fining (bran) tea – use 1 tablespoon of bran per mug, boil and let simmer for 3–5 minutes – fresh vegetable juices, diluted milk, coffee (freshly ground, 1–2 cups a day) with cold-pressed honey.

Assignment

Take hot and cold showers on the spine, 3 minutes hot and 1 minute cold. Finish with a cold one.

CHAPTER 9

The Respiratory System

The functions of the respiratory system are:

- oxygenation
- elimination of carbon dioxide (when too much CO_2 is retained in the blood, the blood turns acidic)
- regulation of acid/base balance of the body

It would benefit many people to learn to breathe properly. Emphasis needs to be placed on emptying the lungs rather than on breathing in. Improved breathing will ensure that carbon monoxide and carbon dioxide are thoroughly expelled from the lungs.

There are four different types of breathing: abdominal, diaphragmatic, intercostal, and clavicular. When you breathe in, the emphasis should be on the neck and the hips going back so that your body adopts a convex posture. Conversely, when breathing out your hips and head should be pushed forward, suggesting a concave posture. Performing 20 full breaths a day would be most beneficial.

Another useful exercise to help open the lungs is to pretend to conduct fast music with two sticks for 5–10 minutes each day.

❄ Diet for asthma

BREAKFAST
A cup of very weak China or Ceylon tea with some honey or a slice of lemon; porridge with molasses, treacle, brown sugar or liquid cold-pressed honey, and dried soaked fruit and an apple (large Bramley) or cereal and fruit or fresh fruit.

LUNCH
Eat raw fruit only such as apples, pears, grapes, plums, kiwi fruit, papaya, custard apples, peaches and rotten bananas.

TEA
A cup of weak tea with a slice of lemon, and a cracker/ryebread (from time to time) with Marmite.

DINNER
Mainly a large vegetable salad, preceded sometimes by soup or a cup of vegetable bouillon, followed by fruit again, usually baked apples or fruit salad – or sometimes a wholewheat steamed fruit pudding, but not often. For a change you may have steamed vegetables of all kinds with baked potatoes, or perhaps an omelette or vegetables or, very occasionally, fish.

- It is very important *not* to eat dairy products because of the amount of mucus that they generate.

❄ Anticatarrhal diet

This diet is therapeutic for common colds and mucus-producing inflammation.

The lungs consist of a number of bronchii. These bronchii divide into bronchioles which further divide into smaller sets of alveoles which absorb the oxygen. If the larger bronchioles close because of inflammation or catarrh, air is unable to enter. A useful exercise to open the lungs is to tap the chest and emit a 'Yaaaii Yaaaii Yaaaii' sound for 3–4 minutes each day.

All plants of the *allium* family are anticatarrhal: chives, onions, garlic, and leeks. Onion soup is a recommended anticatarrhal nutrient. Red onions are more effective than white ones because they are rich in both vitamins A and E. They are also antioxidants. Anticatarrhal food is also hot. Take about 20 peppercorns, put them in the mouth and chew well. Then drink a cup of hot water. It will help to open the lungs.

Menu plan

- Follow this plan as closely as can be managed.
- Drink copious amounts of liquid between meals: water, ginger tea, black tea if desired, and herb tea.
- Eat plenty of fresh figs, oranges, grapes, brown bread, ground almonds, cabbage, spinach, carrots, tomatoes, broccoli and pomegranates.
- Avoid alcohol, all starchy foods, white bread, pastries, white sugar, white flour, sausages, pickles, vinegar, everything that comes out of tins, preserved foods, fried foods.

ON RISING
Drink a glass of warm water containing the juice of a whole lemon or orange, with 1 tablespoon of fructose.

BREAKFAST
Mixed fruit salad, cut up small, with seedless raisins added, and ground or whole nuts; 1 or 2 glasses of diluted fruit juice.

LUNCH
Onion Soup (see below); tomato and green salad; fruit or fruit salad; 1 or 2 slices of brown wholemeal bread with unsalted butter; a glass of fruit juice or instant vegetable bouillon, or 1 teaspoon of Marmite dissolved in a cup of hot water.

DINNER
Broccoli, steamed with some lemon, tamarind and coarse black pepper; 1 type of grain or some potatoes; green salad or raw mixed vegetable salad; as much onion soup as you like; choice of lean meat, fish, or an omelette; pudding made with tapioca or buckwheat.

RECIPE FOR ONION SOUP
Chop the onions, sauté them in a little oil, add water and then boil until half the water has evaporated. Add some paprika, a pinch of salt and some coarse black pepper. Eat it as hot as you can stand it.

Assignments

1 Laugh and sing for at least for 10 minutes in the morning and evening.
2 Go for long walks and talk to the trees.
3 Practise dry skin brushing, remembering to always brush towards the heart.
4 If your nose is clogged up, put a few drops of eucalyptus oil, camphor oil and tea tree oil in a pot with hot water. Put a towel over your head and then inhale the steam to open the bronchial tubes.
5 Have a foot massage to stimulate the lungs.

❋ Dietary treatment of psoriasis and allied skin complaints

As we have seen (pp. 23, 39), the lungs and colon are closely connected. The colon is responsible for the elimination of waste products, but so also is the skin. It is not surprising, therefore, that skin complaints are a by-product of the malfunctioning of the colonic and respiratory systems.

In *psoriasis* a superficial layer of the skin builds up before the old layer is removed. Affected areas are usually elbows, knees and ears. In addition to a strict diet, increased circulation to the skin is helpful. Apply cider vinegar to these vulnerable areas and leave for half an hour, followed by a shower, once a day.

General rules

The following list of forbidden and permissible foodstuffs must be strictly adhered to. Only by scrupulous care with regard to diet for a period of between 9 and 15 months can obstinate cases of skin diseases be driven out of the system. For the first month of treatment a strictly vegetarian diet must be followed. After this initial period, small quantities of fish are permissible for 2 months, followed by a further vegetarian regimen for 1 month, and thereafter 3 months of fish foods, followed by 1 further month of vegetarian food. For the first 3 months of treatment it is imperative to devote 1 whole day per week to eating fruit and drinking fruit juices (see Juice Fast, Chapter 4).

FORBIDDEN
- all fried foods
- beef (in any form), pork, venison, duck, goose, mutton, liver, kidney, heart and sausages – basically, all meat
- oxtail soup, thick meat soups and all tinned or preserved soups
- branded breakfast foods
- preserved meats and meat pastes
- suet and meat puddings
- potatoes (other than baked or boiled in their skins, in small quantities)
- tinned or preserved vegetables and vegetable salads
- thick gravies, chutney, curries, bottled sauces, ordinary salad dressing, common table salt, vinegar, sardines, pickles
- coffee, milk, strong tea, beer, stout, cheap wines

ALLOWED
- biochemical salt
- champagne
- garlic-soaked olives

Assignments

1 Drink 6 cups of echinacea tea a day or mother tincture of echinacea drops – 10 drops in a little water 3 times a day.
2 Have a dry brush body bath once a day.
3 Sing loudly for 10 minutes a day.
4 Take a dip in the Dead Sea for 14 days in a row: that means a trip to Israel! Or use 500g of Dead Sea salt in a bath. Stay in the bath for 30 minutes at a time.

PART II

HEALTH MANUAL

Natural Responses to
Common Ailments

CHAPTER 10

Simple Remedies for Common Ailments

Ill health begins as a number of vague symptoms, followed by discomfort and then dis-ease. Often we ignore these initial symptoms or suppress them by taking an analgesic (pain-killer). In the course of time the untreated dis-ease may well develop into a fully-fledged *disease*. The initial symptoms are a warning that the body is malfunctioning and needs correcting.

In the Health Manual, I document 'natural' responses to many of the more common ailments, listed alphabetically from acne to wrinkles. I recommend a number of 'simple' solutions, mainly – although not exclusively – dietary. Most of the suggested remedies are likely to be found in the kitchen cupboards of the average household.

Body organs

The body is an integrated whole, not a number of disconnected parts as the practices of modern Western medicine might encourage us to believe. The origin of most diseases can be traced to key body organs which have been allowed to malfunction over a period of time. In each section I indicate which malfunctioning organs are causing the disease.

Spinal adjustments

All vertebrae are connected to the body organs via the nervous system, the sympathalic and the parasympathalic. Spinal imbalances influence and may be the cause of some diseases. Chronic spinal imbalances need to be corrected by a professional osteopath or chiropractor. In each section I indicate which vertebrae contribute to the various ailments.

Juices

Some of the most effective remedies are juices made from fresh fruit and raw vegetables. It is advisable to invest in a good quality electric juicer which extracts the maximum amount of juice from fruit and vegetables (the remaining pulp can be used to make stock or soups). All fruit and vegetables should be washed thouroughly, but not skinned or peeled – except bananas, pomegranates, citrus fruits and melons. Include the pips, pith and seeds. All juices are best taken immediately rather than stored in the fridge. They should be sipped slowly while the stomach is empty, preferably first thing in the morning.

Fresh fruit and vegetable juices contain organic acids, which have an alkalizing effect on the body. Most degenerative diseases are the result of excessive acidity, which can be neutralized by the organic acids contained in fruit and vegetables. Fruit juices have a diuretic effect, relieving congestion in the kidneys. They also augment the treatment of arthritis and liver complaints.

In the Fresh Juice Recipes throughout this section, use an *equal amount* of juice from each of the fruits and vegetables listed.

A GOOD GENERAL TONIC
When feeling unwell without any obvious cause, this drink will always be helpful. Make from equal amounts of the following juices:

- carrot
- celery
- cooking apple
- raw beetroot
- parsley

Add a pinch of salt, black pepper and some ground roasted cumin seeds. Drink 500ml, undiluted. Chew 1 slice of fennel root when in season.

In addition, breathe more deeply, emphasizing your out-breaths. Try this exercise for 10 minutes each morning and evening.

If you feel that your system – especially the heart, lungs and liver – is in need of a revitalization programme, try the following:

FRESH JUICE RECIPE

Mix equal amounts of raw beetroot and carrot juice with freshly grated ginger, 1 finely chopped chilli and the pith of a lemon.

Add cayenne pepper and a pinch of salt and black pepper. Drink 1–2 cups first thing every morning.

You should also drink plenty of eucalyptus herb tea and take regular exercise.

❋ Acne

BODY ORGANS
- lungs
- colon
- kidneys

SPINAL ADJUSTMENT
- thoracic 3–4–5–6 and 10–12

VAGUE SYMPTOM STAGE
- itching

DISCOMFORT
- constipation

DIS-EASE
- pimples

DISEASE
- pustules
- boils

Acne usually starts out as a mild rash accompanied by discomfort followed by itching and the appearance of pustules. These are followed by white heads of pus. Squeezing these white heads precipitates spots, which are further worsened by various soaps and creams, often leaving the area infected.

The sebaceous glands in the skin are affected by hormonal disturbances, bad breathing habits and problems with the colon. The colon is the principal cause of skin infection as a result of incomplete elimination.

Once this manifests as acne, it is generally only the symptoms that are treated, not the cause. Treatment needs to be directed to the lungs, colon and kidneys.

The kidneys can disturb the hormonal balance when they malfunction, or the hormones themselves can behave erratically, perhaps as a result of fear. The lungs and colon can fail to function properly through the incomplete elimination of stale air from the lungs and the retention of waste products in the colon. The latter case is often the result of a modern 'junk food' diet.

If you focus on the proper functioning of these organs and maintain a 'clean' body, acne can be made to disappear. But remember, you are treating the whole person, not just the acne symptoms.

The skin

Despite the fact that the skin is the largest of our organs, we tend not to think of it as an organ at all. A key function of the skin is to maintain the temperature of the body. It is also connected directly to the brain. Any waste products which are not eliminated in sputum, urine or faeces are eliminated through the skin.

As an aside, if the skin were completely covered, with paint for instance, a person would live no longer than 3–4 hours. What is also not often realized is that some 90 per cent of the dust in most rooms is skin that has been shed.

Skin manifests a range of characteristics in response to various emotions:

- blue: fear
- goose pimples: happiness
- red, goose pimples: joy
- flushing, heat: anger
- sweat, grey (in chronic cases): apprehension
- green: gall bladder problems, excess bile
- blue, goose pimples: cold
- raised hair: anger and fear

The skin absorbs whatever we apply to it: cosmetics, shampoos, make-up, perfumes. Hydrocortisone is a steroid used to treat inflammatory dermatological conditions such as dermatitis and eczema. It is absorbed via the skin and enters the bloodstream, making its way into various body organs and causing imbalance and damage.

To keep the skin clear, clean out the system regularly with the following juice:

FRESH JUICE RECIPE
Mix together equal amounts of the following juices to make 375ml.

- carrot
- celery
- cucumber
- grape
- raw potato (with skin)

Add 125ml of spring water, a pinch each of salt, black pepper, cumin powder and paprika. Sip slowly on an empty stomach 3 times a week.

❃ Anaemia

BODY ORGANS
- bonemarrow
- spleen
- kidneys

SPINAL ADJUSTMENT
- lumbar area

VAGUE SYMPTOMS
- lack of energy
- palor
- dull eyes
- fatigue
- lethargy
- difficulty in running and breathing

DISCOMFORT
- wounds take longer to heal
- cramps
- indigestion
- insomnia

DIS-EASE:
- halitosis
- strong smelling urine

Anaemia indicates that there is insufficient haemoglobin in the body. Ferrum (iron) pills are not a general solution because they cause constipation. I recommend instead homoeopathic tissue salts Ferr. Phos. D6. (This treatment – referred to hereafter as 'tissue salts' – was originated by Dr Schuessler in the last century and has since gained a world-wide reputation for its effectiveness in stimulating blood circulation and cell reproduction.) Or eat beetroot to stimulate movement in your bowels; it is a healthier solution. If there is a haemolytic disease in the body – you will need a blood test to check – then this treatment is insufficient.

Provided that your anaemia is not pernicious and you have no other chronic blood disease, the following juice will be helpful.

FRESH JUICE RECIPE
Make 375ml from equal amounts of the following juices:

- carrot
- raw beetroot
- celery
- spinach

Add 125ml of spring water with a pinch each of salt, ground black pepper and ground roasted cumin seeds. Cumin powder is very digestible and helps to balance the beetroot which is very earthy and difficult to digest. Chewing 25g of parsley will maximize the effect of this juice, which you should drink twice a day.

In addition, eat mackerel, oysters, sardines, walnuts and broccoli, which are all rich in zinc. Try to eat more green vegetables; they are rich in chlorophyll and will help generally.

❋ Angina pectoris

BODY ORGANS
- spleen
- stomach

- liver
- gall bladder

SPINAL ADJUSTMENT
- thoracic 1–2, 4–10 and cervical 4–5–6–7

VAGUE SYMPTOMS
- burping
- tightness in the chest
- tingling in the little finger

DISCOMFORT
- lethargy
- dry mouth
- heavy head
- constipation

DIS-EASE
- high cholesterol
- dysfunction of small intestines

Angina pectoris can develop over a long period of time with only the vaguest of symptoms. By the time it has been diagnosed, your digestive system will have suffered much abuse. Overloading the digestive system puts significant pressure on the heart muscles. Sudden angina can be triggered by stress, shocks, overeating or bad breathing habits. Angina pectoris manifests as a shooting pain in the chest.

Provided that angina pectoris is not due specifically to digestive problems and you have no ulcers or chronic heart disease, I recommend the following juice.

FRESH JUICE RECIPE
Make 375ml from equal amounts of the following juices:
- carrot
- celery
- spinach

In 500ml of water boil 25g hawthorn berries and 25g lily of the valley leaves until 125ml is left. When cooled add to the fresh juice. Drink twice a day until symptoms abate.

❊ Angry liver

SPINAL ADJUSTMENT
- thoracic 4–5

VAGUE SYMPTOMS
- red eyes
- bitter taste in the mouth
- short temper
- post-alcoholic nausea first thing in the morning

DISCOMFORT
- slight pressure on the right side where the liver is located
- indigestion and constipation

The following juice will give the liver a good cleanse.

FRESH JUICE RECIPE
Make 375ml from equal amounts of the following juices:
- cooking apple
- celery
- carrot

Then prepare a mixture by boiling 2 tablespoons of dried dandelion leaves and root (from a herbalist), with a pinch each of powdered clove, salt and cinnamon, in 500ml of water until 125ml is left. Add the mixture to the juice. Drink while chewing 25g of fresh parsley – on an empty stomach, once or twice a day.

❊ Arthritis

BODY ORGANS
- stomach
- kidneys

SPINAL ADJUSTMENT
- lower lumbar

VAGUE SYMPTOMS
- aches and pains in various places

DISCOMFORT
• difficulty in bending and stretching

Generically, arthritis refers to inflammation of the bones. There are a number of forms: rheumatoid arthritis, osteoarthritis and rheumatoid spondylitis, to name just a few, but rheumatoid arthritis is probably the most painful.

Arthritis is caused by an over-production of acid which is deposited in the joints in the form of crystals. Treatment aims to completely eliminate these crystals without causing damage to the body. I recommend a potato peel diet.

REMEDY
Boil 1kg of 12mm-thick potato peelings in 3½ litres of water. Mash them and eat nothing else for at least 7 days, drinking lots of hot water at the same time. This diet provides dramatic, sudden relief. Avoid aspirin-based tablets during this period. Follow this diet by eating only raw food for 28 days. The two diets should relieve the acute pain and result in the body functioning more effectively.

After the two diets (7 days and 28 days), continue to eat only non-protein food. If you require protein, eat only vegetable proteins such as lentils, legumes and soya beans. Avoid eating eggs, poultry and, most definitely, red meat. If your desire for protein proves irresistible eat sea fish, but avoid the scavengers such as prawns, shrimps and shellfish.

It is advisable to consult a medical practitioner before commencing this diet and allow him or her to supervise you during the 5 weeks of self-treatment.

In addition to the above diets, the discomfort of arthritis can be further minimized by taking hot baths containing 500g of Epsom salts, 500g of sea salt and 125g of bicarbonate of soda. Having the bath as hot as you can bear it for 20–30 minutes, adding hot water every 5 minutes, enables all the pores to open fully. Follow this bath with a cold shower to close the pores. Go directly to bed after drying the body. The sweating will help dispel excessive acid from the body.

While osteoarthritis is difficult to treat with juices, rheumatoid arthritis can certainly be helped during the early stages.

FRESH JUICE RECIPE
Make 500ml from equal amounts of the following juices:
- carrot
- celery
- raw beetroot
- cucumber (with skin)

Drink undiluted on an empty stomach and at the same time chew and eat 100g of ripe pineapple.

Prevention

The best way to prevent a chronic disease such as arthritis is to ensure that you eat balanced meals. An effective diet contains 80 per cent alkaline-forming and 20 per cent acid-forming foods. Remember the general rule – food that is acid/sour before eating becomes alkaline when digested. Most vegetables and fruits are alkaline-forming. Berries are acid-forming. Grains are acid-forming with the exception of millet. Fizzy drinks, coffee, black tea and beverages are all acid-forming. Water, fresh fruit and vegetables, juices and herb teas are alkaline-forming. This diet has a pre-ventative effect; try it from time to time if you are prone to arthritis.

❊ Athlete's foot

BODY ORGANS
- lungs
- colon

SPINAL ADJUSTMENT
- lumbar plexus, lumbar 2–5, thoracic 3–4–5, cervical 1–4

Eat 500g of ripe plums for breakfast for 21 days. This diet will stimulate and cleanse the colon. It will also have an effect on the lungs and improve breathing.

- Change your socks every day. The material should be pure wool, cotton or silk.
- Do not wear the same shoes more than once every 3 days.
- Wear leather soles for 1 year (no rubber soles during this period).

– Wash your feet and toes each evening with 1 teaspoon of cider vinegar
  added to a cup of water.
– Dab each toe with liquid honey, bandage and keep on overnight.

Avoid powder on the feet, rubber shoes for 3–5 years, red meat, hydrocortisone or betnovate creams.

❋ Back pain

The main causes of back pain are:
- neck or hip out of alignment
- malfunctioning kidneys
- bad body posture
- lifting heavy items

BODY ORGANS
- kidneys (lower back)
- gall bladder and intestines (between the shoulders),
- lungs (upper back)

SPINAL ADJUSTMENT
- in the related areas

VAGUE SYMPTOMS
- itching
- soreness
- strong smelling urine
- constipation
- desire for salty foods
- insufficient urination

DISCOMFORT
- pain in back/shoulder muscles
- stiff muscles

General back pain

– Take hot baths with a handful of Epsom salts added, followed by a cold
  shower.

– Have Alexander technique lessons to correct your body posture.
– Take a barley drink to strengthen the kidneys. To 3 litres of water add a cup of barley, 6 peppercorns, 6 cloves, 40 juniper berries, 6 cinnamon sticks and 6 cardamoms (black for men, white for women). Boil down to 1½ litres. Drink this preparation each day for 3 days if the pain persists.
– Put a ginger compress on the painful area (see Appendix B).
– Drink white willow bark tea.

Upper back pain

– Eat onions to strengthen the lungs.
– Hang from a cross-bar with everted then inverted hands.
– Alternate cold and hot water on the spine for 3 minutes, ending with a cold shower.

REMEDIES
– Crush 40 ice cubes. Place directly on the skin in the painful area. Cover with a towel. Repeat twice a day. There are 5 stages: wet, cold, painful, burning, numbness. This treatment takes 20–30 minutes. Remove ice when numbness occurs.

– Mix 1 part wintergreen oil, 1 part tea tree oil and 1 part lavender oil. Add 3 parts olive oil. Shake well before applying to the painful area. Rub in gently. This will increase the healing process. Try not to take pain killers; they can cause constipation and harm the digestive system.

– Take the following vitamins: DLPA 375, PABA 500, Pantothenic Acid 500, Zinc B13 – 1 tablet of each twice a day after meals.

– Have hot baths and cold showers on the spine. Continue for 14 days.

✳ Boils and carbuncles

Symptoms and discomfort are similar to those described for Acne. The main organs involved are the lungs and colon. Boils and carbuncles also appear when the blood is impure, in which case treatment needs to be directed at the liver (see Angry Liver).

REMEDY
Put a poultice of baked onions on the boil or carbuncle; bandage and leave overnight.

The following drink will help to cleanse the colon and lungs.

FRESH JUICE RECIPE
Make 500ml from equal amounts of these juices:
- carrot
- raw beetroot
- spinach
- cucumber

Add a pinch of salt, ½ teaspoon paprika and ¼ teaspoon turmeric. Drink *undiluted* 3 times a day when stomach is empty.

❈ Breathing problems

BODY ORGANS
- lungs
- colon

SPINAL ADJUSTMENT
- upper cervical 1–4 and thoracic 5–7

Many people with breathing difficulties believe that their problem is one of inhalation. I suggest that the problem is rather one of exhalation. Most people use only one-third of their lungs, retaining stale air. They attempt to inhale more air before the stale air has been completely expelled.

Asthmatic people often become anxious and gasp for breath before having emptied their lungs. They are well advised to seek training in how to breathe properly. A change of diet could also have a beneficial effect.

- Limit your intake of fatty foods and proteins, particularly animal proteins.
- Eat mainly fruit, vegetables and minerals.
- Minimize your intake of milk and dairy products, sugar and wheat products, particularly if you show any allergy to the latter.
- Consult an allergy specialist or nutritionist. Discover the foods to which

your body is tolerant and eat only those foods for one whole year, through all four seasons, until your body has cleared itself.
– Eat onions and onion soups. Onions are anticatarrhal.

Simple tissue salts and combination tissue salts are available for specific ailments. If you suffer an acute attack with extreme difficulty in breathing, try one of the following acidic drinks to relieve the tension inside your body.

• cider vinegar
• lemon and honey
• effervescent vitamin C

Apart from the above advice, the most effective remedy is controlled breathing and posture. Proper body adjustment with the help of an osteopath will help to relax the body. I also recommend breathing exercises and yoga.

✳ Bruises

BODY ORGANS
• spleen
• liver
• pancreas
• chest bone
• thymus

SPINAL ADJUSTMENT
• thoracic 4–9

Bruises result from a lack of vitamin K, bad circulation and the excessive use of hydrocortisone. To correct the vitamin deficiency, include the following in your diet:
– Pumpkin seeds. They are rich in vitamin K and zinc and also function as a laxative. Eat 100–200g a day for at least 6 months.
– Watercress. It is rich in vitamin K (anti-coagulant). Ensure that you clean the roots thoroughly and that no fungus remains.

- Seaweed. It is an antioxidant, rich in minerals and chlorophyll
- Watercress, cabbage, broccoli and cauliflower. These cruciferous plants are antioxidant and rich in zinc and sulphur.

❋ Burns

Burns are described according to their severity – first-, second- or third-degree. Regardless of the degree of burn, Arnica D6 taken internally will help counteract shock.

A slight burn which reddens the skin is a first-degree burn. This could be the result of sunburn or of having touched something hot. In order to take the heat out of the skin, direct application of potato peel, yoghurt, witch hazel or bicarbonate of soda dissolved in water is effective.

A second-degree burn is more serious, with burns over a larger area of skin. The most effective initial response is to apply running water for about 10 minutes, and then apply crushed ice. It is important that the ice is placed directly on the skin and not put in a plastic bag. Leave the ice in place until the whole area feels numb. This will take at least 20 minutes.

Do not apply any creams. They protect the skin with a cover and in so doing prevent the heat from leaving the skin, which will then blister. It would be more effective to cover the burnt area with bioyoghurt. Leave it in place until the pain has completely dispersed. It may be necessary to change the yoghurt once or twice. If the burn is very serious, apply cool tofu and cover with a bandage. When the tofu becomes warm, change the bandage. Should the burn leave an open wound, apply cold-pressed natural honey. The honey-covered wound can be covered with a plaster for 48 hours. Avoid water coming into contact with the affected area. This treatment will usually not leave any scars. Vitamin E capsules will help the fragile skin to heal and strengthen. Open the capsules and apply the oil directly to the skin.

A third-degree burn is very serious. It means that the burnt area is large and the person is in a state of shock. The affected area can be treated with pure, cold-pressed liquid honey. Ensure that the burnt area is not wet. It is essential to seek medical help.

❋ Catarrh

BODY ORGANS
- lungs
- colon

SPINAL ADJUSTMENT
- cervical 1–4 and thoracic 2–3–5

VAGUE SYMPTOMS
- sore throat
- sneezing

DISCOMFORT
- watery nose
- swollen glands
- difficulties with swallowing
- coughing

DIS-EASE
- sinusitis
- bronchitis
- angina
- rhinitis
- influenza

When antibiotics are taken to destroy catabolic bacteria they also injure the anabolic bacteria that are essential for various bodily functions.

For a better, natural remedy:

- Chew 20 peppercorns (at the same time, not one at a time) and drink a cup of hot water. Repeat this exercise every 4 hours over a 48-hour period (during waking hours only). The catarrh should clear provided there is no other medical problem.
- Eat plenty of onions or onion soup, both of which contain vitamins C and E. Onions are the ultimate anticatarrhal vegetable.
- Minimize fatty foods and drink as much water as possible.

If the symptoms do not clear up after about 3 days, consult a medical practitioner, naturopath or nutritionist.

The following drink will help cleanse and strengthen the colon and lungs, and aid elimination:

FRESH JUICE RECIPE
Make 500ml from equal amounts of the following juices:
- carrot
- spinach
- raw beetroot
- cucumber

Add a pinch each of salt, black pepper and paprika. Drink undiluted twice a day. At the same time chew 2 cloves of garlic.

❋ Cholesterol problems

BODY ORGANS
- gall bladder
- liver

SPINAL ADJUSTMENT
- thoracic 3–4 and 10

The levels of high and low density lipoproteins (HDL and LDL) need to be viewed in contrast to each other. Neither is useful as an indicator on its own. HDL should always be high and LDL should be low.

From a natural health perspective, a high level of cholesterol in the blood suggests extreme unresolved anger as well as shallow breathing habits. The following remedies would help to normalize cholesterol levels.

- Practise expelling all the air from your lungs.
- Drink 25ml of safflower oil before going to bed.
- Eat lots of onions in any form, preferably red onions.
- Eat more natural foods, raw food in particular.

❋ Colds

BODY ORGANS
- lungs
- colon
- immune system

SPINAL ADJUSTMENT
- cervical 1–4 and thoracic 3–4–5

A cold is actually your friend rather than your enemy. It is the body's response to foreign invasion. The acute production of fluids is its way of expelling the invaders. The important point to note is that even before your cold develops, your immune system has become so debilitated that the invaders see your body as a benign environment. Antibiotics will certainly help to expel these enemies, but they will not alter your body's benign status. The more sensible and longer-term approach is to render your body hostile to interlopers.

Antibiotics furthermore can have a negative effect on the body generally. A more natural and balanced way to respond to colds might be as follows:

- Tone up your body with a hot bath followed by a cold shower.
- Eat more anticatarrhal foods such as onions, garlic, chives, ginger (food that is hot, bitter, putrid or astringent rather than sweet, sour or salty).
- Drink hot lemon and honey (as effective a cure for colds as any medicine dispensed by a chemist).
- The most effective relief for a really rough throat combined with a cold is to eat 20 peppercorns (at the same time, not one at a time). It may seem dramatic, but it works. Chew them and drink a cup of hot water. The relief is usually immediate. If you continue to be plagued, repeat every 4 hours.
- If your cold is accompanied by constipation and you do not have onions or cannot make soup, buy effervescent vitamin C tablets. Take 2 in a glass of water every 2 hours until bowel movement begins. Should diarrhoea set in, this will indicate that your cold has been dispelled.

The popular myth that you should starve a fever and feed a cold is incorrect. The opposite is the case. Starve the cold and feed the fever. When

you have a fever the body needs energy to fight it. It should be fed slowly.
 I recommend the following additional remedies for a sore throat.

– a 24-hour fast
– Olbas oil lozenges
– a gargle made with sage, or a rind of lemon if no sage is available. Squeeze the juice out of the lemon, grate the rind and boil in water.

FRESH JUICE RECIPE
Mix together equal amounts of the following juices to make 750ml:

- lemon
- carrot
- grapefruit
- orange

Add 250ml of spring water and a pinch each of salt and black pepper. Drink while chewing on a piece of fresh ginger

❉ Colds, coughs and fevers

For a fast remedy, mix together the juice of 1 onion with the juice of 1 lemon. Drink the mixture followed by a cup of hot water.

❉ Colitis (inflammation of the colon)

ORGAN
- colon

SPINAL ADJUSTMENT
- sacrum

VAGUE SYMPTOMS
- belching
- gas

DISCOMFORT
- pain on the right side of the solar plexus
- constipation alternating with diarrhoea

DIS-EASE
- the stomach is over-producing acid
- the pancreas is under-producing pancreatic juices and not having a neutralizing effect

DISEASE
- mucus in stools
- spastic pain and cramps
- intolerance of food
- gas, distention and bloating
- occasional blood in stools

Provided there is no blood in the stools and no history of alternating constipation and diarrhoea, the following juice should be taken 3–4 times a day.

FRESH JUICE RECIPE

Make 500ml from equal amounts of the following juices:
- carrot
- cooking apple
- raw beetroot
- cucumber

Drink undiluted with a pinch each of salt, black pepper and ground roasted cumin seeds.

Avoid preserved and tinned food.

❋ Colon (infection of)

BODY ORGANS
- colon
- small intestines

SPINAL ADJUSTMENT
- thoracic 6–7–8

DIS-EASE
- bloated abdomen and gas
- pain in the abdomen when it is bloated
- bad breath in the morning

REMEDIES

For breakfast eat 1 head of cos lettuce, mixed with 100g of bioyoghurt to soothe the stomach. Eat more barley, oats and rice. Cut out wheat, cheese, red meat. Eat raw food during the day. In the evening eat over-cooked brown rice, undercooked vegetables with umeboshi plums and as much fish as you can manage. Avoid lentils – they produce wind. Arrange to have colonic irrigation, performed preferably by a practitioner who has been personally recommended.

Drink a tea made of:
- 1 litre water
- 1 teaspoon ginger
- 1 stick cinnamon
- 6 cloves

Boil for 5 minutes and drink 1 cup 3 times a day.

❋ Congested nose

SPINAL ADJUSTMENT
- cervical 1–4

Reasons for congestion
- polyps have grown in the nasal passages
- the tissue attached to the turbinate bones in the nasal passages is swollen (they have erectile cells which react to emotions)

If you have chronic breathing problems at night:
- Place 1 teaspoon salt in a glass of water and sniff in through the nose to clean out the sinuses.
- Rub a drop of cold-pressed sesame oil into the nasal passages with your finger.

✳ Constipation

BODY ORGANS
- colon
- lungs
- gall bladder, sometimes (too much bile causes diarrhoea whilst too little causes constipation)

PSYCHOLOGICAL ASPECTS
- miserliness
- holding on/tight-fisted
- not letting go

EMOTIONAL ASPECT
- apprehension

If you are constipated you are not emptying your bowels properly. In the process of evacuation you initially pass water, followed by stools. A sign that the bowels have emptied is a second passing of water. If this does not occur then your bowels are not completely empty. Drinking lots of water will clear constipation in most cases.

From a psychological perspective, constipated people can be regarded as misers. They are trying to hold onto things, including their own waste. I encourage my constipated patients to get rid of an object that they have not used in the past five years so that they can begin to think in terms of 'letting go'. This often results in the bowels moving again.

Many people take laxatives. Habitual use of laxatives forces the body to perform its necessary functions unnaturally. Laxatives are quite unnecessary if you can eat sufficient roughage and drink enough water. The natural way to overcome the problem is to eat foods which have a naturally laxative effect – such as onion soup, pears, plums, bran, linseed oil, green vegetables and minerals – and avoid starchy foods and white flour products.

Diet suggestion

BREAKFAST
- 2 tablespoons of bran
- 2 tablespoons of linseed oil mixed with 1 rotten overripe black banana

- orange juice or apple juice

LUNCH AND DINNER
- eat green vegetables rather than root vegetables
- eliminate starchy puddings
- drink sufficient water to flush your system

The colon can quite easily be restored to normal functioning within 21–28 days. Insufficient exercise combined with long periods of sitting can often cause constipation because of the lack of movement. If your work is sedentary, you can help yourself by performing regular abdominal exercises. Singing is also most helpful.

FRESH JUICE RECIPE
Make 500ml from equal amounts of the following juices:
- carrot
- cooking apple
- spinach
- grape

Drink undiluted on an empty stomach. Add a pinch of salt and black pepper and eat 1 raw courgette. While drinking this juice, practise 'eating the drink'.

Chronic constipation

From time to time fast for 24 hours, drinking only warm water.

RECIPE
- 100g almonds (skinned)
- 2 cardamoms (small)
- 1 tablespoon jaggery
- 1 tablespoon poppy seeds
- 4 cups soya curd milk
- 25g pork fat

Grind the ingredients into a paste and fry together. Drink slowly and the bowels will move within half an hour. Jaggery is unrefined sugar from sugar cane and can be obtained from most Asian foodstores. If you cannot buy soya curd milk, you can make it yourself in the same way as you would make yoghurt from cow's milk. Soya bean milk can be purchased from most healthfood stores and large supermarkets.

❄ Coughs

BODY ORGANS
- lungs
- colon

SPINAL ADJUSTMENT
- cervical 1–4 and thoracic 3–4–5–6

SYMPTOMS
- itching of the throat
- irritation inside the larynx

It is important to find the cause of a cough. It could be a cold, glandular swelling, influenza, or something you have eaten that has irritated your system. Once the cause has been found it can be treated. In the meantime, you can relieve the cough itself by gargling with sage, eucalyptus oil, lemon and honey or by applying glycerine and bicarbonate of soda to the throat.

If the irritation is removed, the cough will subside. But if the cough is the secondary effect of something else, it is necessary to deal with the primary cause, rather than suppress the cough. One of the best ways to tone up the body is to take hot baths followed by cold showers. Also, eat more antioxidants such as onions, garlic, chives and ginger.

If the symptoms do not clear up after about 3 days, consult a medical practitioner, naturopath or nutritionist.

COUGH SYRUP
- Cover 250g of small onions (chopped) with honey, cinnamon and cloves. Simmer in a pan for 3–5 minutes and eat before going to bed.

MIXTURE FOR A CHRONIC COUGH
- 1 teaspoon grated ginger
- 1 teaspoon grated garlic
- 1 teaspoon grated red onion

Add 3 teaspoons of honey, mix and leave for 24 hours. Take ½ teaspoon in the morning and evening for 7 days.

❋ Cystitis (bladder infection)

ORGAN
- bladder

SPINAL ADJUSTMENT
- lumbar 1–5 and sacrum

ACUTE SYMPTOMS
- blood in urine
- pain in the urethra

DISCOMFORT
- chill
- burning sensation in the bladder and on passing urine (men only)

Cystitis is just as likely to be caused by a chill as by excessive consumption of a particular kind of alcohol. An attack occurs when the urethras – tubes that lead from the kidneys to the bladder – become inflamed. Infection also can be communicated to the kidneys from the colon.

It is important to drink as much liquid as possible. I recommend:

- 1 teaspoon finely grated lemon rind – not the juice
- 1 teaspoon ground cinnamon

Boil in 1½ litres of water and drink while hot. If no lemon or cinnamon is available, use cranberry juice, but you must warm it first.

If you are unable to find the above ingredients, drink sage or camomile tea in the meantime.

The following barley soup can also be most helpful.

- 6 cinnamon sticks
- 6 cloves
- 6 cardamoms (black for men, white for women)
- 40 juniper berries
- 1 teaspoon fennel seeds
- 1 cup barley
- 3 litres water

Boil the concoction down to 1½ litres – filter and consume while hot.

Eat no protein of any kind and eat vegetables and fruit exclusively for 48 hours. Healthfood stores can usually recommend specific herbal teas and tissue salts for cystitis.

FRESH JUICE RECIPE

Make 500ml from equal amounts of the following juices:

- carrot
- spinach
- parsley
- raw beetroot
- cucumber

Add a pinch each of salt, black pepper, cinnamon and ground roasted cumin seeds. Drink undiluted. Eat 1 pomegranate or 500g of watermelon while doing so. It is also helpful if you chew the seeds of the pomegranate and watermelon.

❊ Diarrhoea

BODY ORGANS

- lungs
- liver
- colon

SPINAL ADJUSTMENT

- thoracic 3–4–5–6, lumbar 1–5 and sacrum

Diarrhoea is nature's way of getting rid of food which your system has reacted to. It is therefore a cure rather than an illness.

The best commonly available remedy is very soft white bread, preferably freshly baked. Take the inside from a loaf and roll into 10–15 small balls of 2.5cm diameter. Dip the balls into live yoghurt and swallow without chewing. This should stop the diarrhoea immediately.

Another effective remedy is fenugreek powder. Use 1 teaspoon of the powder mixed into a cup of water. Drink 2–3 cups.

A third cure to stop diarrhoea is apples. Remove the skin and cores, chop finely and boil in a little water. Eat nothing else for 24 hours and do not take any drugs or you will suffer the reverse effect – constipation.

Drink carbonated (fizzy) drinks, mint tea, camomile tea, or watercress tea. Boil chopped up watercress in water and drink. The sulphur in watercress is particularly beneficial. It purifies the blood and is effective in clearing out the system and strengthening the liver.

I can also recommend charcoal tablets, known in homoeopathy as Carbo. veg.

A final more general remedy consists of mixing 1 teaspoon of finely grated ginger with 20 drops of soy sauce in a cup of hot water

If the diarrhoea does not stop within 24 hours after you have tried one or more of the above cures, consider seeking professional assistance.

FRESH JUICE RECIPE
Make 375ml from equal amounts of the following juices:
- carrot
- celery
- spinach
- parsley
- raspberry (from fresh or frozen fruit)

Boil 1 tablespoon dried blackberries (from herbalist) in 500ml of water until 125ml remains. Add a pinch of salt and nutmeg and 1 level teaspoon fenugreek powder. Mix with the juice and drink 1–1½ litres a day.

❋ Earache

BODY ORGANS
- kidneys

SPINAL ADJUSTMENT
- cervical 1–2–3–4

VAGUE SYMPTOMS AND DISCOMFORT
- itching in the ear
- discomfort in earlobe
- nasal congestion
- pressure behind the earlobe

Apart from draughts or a blockage, the cause of earache is generally an infection of the Eustachian tube, which links the throat and the ear. It is, however, important to ensure that the inside of the ear is not clogged.

The most effective way to clean the ears is with a 2 per cent solution of hydrogen peroxide. Insert 2 drops into the ear, let it bubble and clean out with a soft swab. Then plug the ear with 1 drop of sesame oil, at or around room temperature. The sesame oil should be unrefined, pure, unheated oil.

Try an anticatarrhal diet, such as chives, garlic, red (not white) onions, mustard cress, horseradish, ordinary mustard and endives. Although endives are very rich and bitter, they are also anticatarrhal.

For older people with earache, I recommend the following. Heat a stone or half a brick in the oven. Then wrap it in a towel and hold it against the ear. Remove it if the heat is intolerable and replace against the ear when it has cooled slightly. This dry heat treatment, unlike a hot water bottle, will help to reduce the earache.

✳ Eczema

BODY ORGANS
- lungs
- colon

SPINAL ADJUSTMENT
- thoracic 5–8, lumbar 2–5 and sacrum

VAGUE SYMPTOMS
- scratching
- skin discoloration

DISCOMFORT
- rash from washing powder, solvents or detergents
- pain from tick bites

DISEASE
- oozing
- aberration

Eczema is a common word for different forms of skin irritation. It can describe eczema caused by environmental conditions, skin rash or heat eczema. The skin should be acidic and not alkaline. If it is too alkaline it becomes hospitable to various diseases.

In order to increase the acidity of the skin, bath with Epsom salts (magnesium sulphate). Or pour a cup of organic cider vinegar into the bath. Also use less soap. Buy pH-neutral products. Experiment with different washing detergents and ensure that you do not touch them with your bare hands.

The skin is directly connected to the lungs and assists in the breathing process. When you fail to breathe properly through the lungs the skin will try to eliminate what the lungs and colon have failed to expel.

Many people who have breathing problems are apprehensive. Learn to relax and breathe out more effectively, expelling the carbon monoxide and carbon dioxide from your system. Cleansing the system generally will assist to cleanse away the eczema.

Find out if you have used any creams which contain hydrocortisone, which could well still be in your system. These are best eliminated by an effective diet or fast. External relief can be gained from cream that contains vitamins A, D and E, echinecea or cassia cream, but check it does *not* contain any hydrocortisone.

If the eczema causes oozing with itching and pus, consult a physician.

✳ Excess weight

BODY ORGANS
- gall bladder
- liver
- stomach
- pancreas
- kidneys

SPINAL ADJUSTMENT
- entire lumbar area

EMOTIONAL ASPECTS
- fear
- apprehension

Fat provides the body with warmth and is therefore a comfort factor. But it is unhealthy. Unless there is a glandular problem, overweight people have a clear need for a low-fat diet using unsaturated polyacids and cold-pressed oils rather than animal fats.

Many overweight people are fat because they eat to give themselves a feeling of being full. They have a need to feel that they have *really* eaten.

Prevention

– Eat when hungry, not by the clock.
– Eat sitting down: no reading, speaking, or telephone calls.
– Eat more pungent, hot, putrid, astringent, bitter foods.
– Cut down on sweet, sour, salty foods.
– Eat to satisfy half your hunger and avoid starch where possible.
– Eat starch with minerals, proteins with minerals, and fat with minerals.
– Do not eat starch with protein and do not eat starch with fat as a general rule. But do not become over-idiosyncratic. Remember, all foods contain proteins, fats, carbohydrates and minerals. It is only their proportions that vary.

FRESH JUICE RECIPE
Combine equal amounts of the following juices:
• carrot
• celery
• spinach
• cucumber

Drink 2–3 litres a day, undiluted. Chew celery or a courgette while drinking the juice.

❋ Eye problems

BODY ORGANS
• liver
• thymus
• kidneys
• spleen

SPINAL ADJUSTMENT
• entire cervical area and mid-dorsal

VAGUE SYMPTOMS
• itching
• grinding eyes
• red eyes
• strain from light, reading, overwork, computer screens

DISCOMFORT
- blurred vision
- night blindness
- boil on eyelids

These problems are generally due to a vitamin deficiency, particularly of vitamins A and B.

FRESH JUICE RECIPE
Make 500ml from equal amounts of the following juices:
- carrot
- celery
- parsley

Add a pinch of salt and black pepper, and ½ teaspoon paprika or 10 drops of tabasco. Drink undiluted.

Eye inflammation

PSYCHOLOGICAL ASPECT
- unwillingness to see

EMOTIONAL ASPECT
- anger

The eyes are linked to the liver. The emotion of the liver is anger. When anger is repressed, it can result in inflammation. Eyes can express considerable anger. It would be helpful to learn to express your anger. Try shadow boxing for 10 minutes every day. When fear blocks anger, the result is an excess of mucus and inflammations in eyes and ears, so try to express your fear.

- Eat olives in soaked garlic to clean the liver – available from most delicatessens.
- Drink 500ml of freshly made carrot juice a day.
- Use midstream urine for an eye-bath, then put honey on the eye, cover and sleep with it in place (an unusual treatment, but effective).
- Try euphrasia eye drops from a homoeopathic store for a slight eye infection.

❋ Flatulence

BODY ORGANS
• colon

SPINAL ADJUSTMENT
• not needed

There are many ways to avoid flatulence. Chronic flatulence or belching
is the result of fermentation in the small and large intestines. It can occur
because you have swallowed too much air; your fermentation process is
out of balance (the result of an excess of magnesium and a deficiency of
sodium and calcium in your food); you have eaten too fast; or you are ill.

REMEDIES
– Take a cup of hot water and add 1 teaspoon of cider. Sit down when you
  drink it and avoid activities for a while.
– Drink a cup of celery juice.
– Take the juice of ½ lemon, 1 teaspoon of honey and add hot water.
– Be silent when eating to avoid swallowing air. Chew food thoroughly.
– Use asafoetida in lentils when cooking.
– Cook lentils without salt until they are overcooked, glutinous and slimy.
  Salt can be added to spicy lentil dishes afterwards; otherwise they will
  produce flatulence.

❋ Fungal infections

BODY ORGANS
• lungs
• colon

SPINAL ADJUSTMENT
• thoracic 2–3

During the summer fungus is often found in moist parts of the body – the
scrotum, anus, armpits or chest. It forms reddish spots accompanied by
itching.

REMEDIES
- Put 10 drops of bleach in 500ml of water, mix and sponge your body until all the liquid is used up.
- Use tea tree oil on the affected area (it takes longer to work, but also has antiseptic values).
- Use a purgative to clean the colon.
- Perform breathing exercises to clean the lungs.

FRESH JUICE RECIPE
Make 500ml from equal amounts of the following juices:
- carrot
- spinach
- beetroot
- cucumber

Add a pinch of salt and black pepper, and ½ teaspoon paprika. Drink undiluted. Eat a carrot while drinking.

✳ Gout

BODY ORGANS
- liver
- kidneys
- colon

SPINAL ADJUSTMENT
- entire thoracic area

VAGUE SYMPTOMS
- swollen toe
- pain when putting pressure on the foot
- bitter taste in the mouth

DISCOMFORT
- inability to walk as a result of pain in the feet or knees

This disease is caused by an excess of uric acid in the blood. It usually affects one of the big toes.

FRESH JUICE RECIPE
Make 500ml from equal amounts of the following juices:

- carrot
- celery
- spinach
- cucumber (with skin)

Add a pinch each of salt, black pepper, ground roasted cumin seeds and the juice of 1 lemon. Drink undiluted. Eat 2 slices of fresh overripe pineapple while drinking this juice.

❈ Gum and tooth disorders

BODY ORGANS
- stomach – lower teeth
- colon – upper teeth

SPINAL ADJUSTMENT
- lumbar 1–5, sacrum and thoracic 6–12

Clove oil is a wonderful anaesthetic, especially when your gums are painful. Use a cotton swab or, in an emergency, a matchstick covered with material. Dip the swab into the clove oil and apply to the painful area. If it is of sufficient strength the clove oil will numb the nerve. If it penetrates, it may well take the pain out of the gum. This is not a cure, but will provide temporary relief from toothache. Failure to properly clean the oral cavity will leave bacteria in place and result in the return of the infection. If you cannot obtain clove oil, use cloves. Chew them or put them onto the painful tooth and bite. This should provide some relief.

If the gums are very swollen, use the following remedy:

- ½ teaspoon of bicarbonate of soda
- ½ teaspoon of salt
- 2 drops of mustard oil

Apply the mixture to the entire mouth, letting it flow over the gums. Ensure that you visit a dentist and oral hygienist as soon as possible.

Dental hygiene is best achieved by avoiding substances that are rich in sugar, such as sweets, lozenges and chocolates. Try to finish meals with an apple, particularly if you are unable to brush your teeth. Apples are good cleaners for the teeth and gums. Brush your teeth at least twice a day, on waking and before going to bed. Massage the gums regularly with a finger.

Disorders of the lower teeth suggest a stomach disorder and the need for more alkaline-forming food. Infection of the upper teeth suggests a disorder of the colon, which can be cleaned with the following juice.

FRESH JUICE RECIPE
Make 500ml from equal amounts of the following juices:
- celery
- spinach
- raw beetroot
- cooking apple

Add a pinch of salt and black pepper and ½ teaspoon of paprika. Drink undiluted. Chew 25g of parsley while drinking this juice.

❋ Haemorrhoids

BODY ORGANS
- colon

SPINAL ADJUSTMENT
- lumbar 3–4–5 and coccyx

Haemorroids are caused by a faulty valve in the veins in the lower bowel; the veins then swell with blood and form grapes. When the bowels do not move and pressure in the abdomen blocks the blood circulation, trouble begins.

Prevention

Avoid constipation. Each day eat 1 tablespoon of psyllium husks and add 1 teaspoon of slippery elm to a cold drink to keep the bowels moving.

Sometimes haemorrhoids are caused by asthma, bronchitis or other stresses in the body. They can be either external (in the anus area) or internal (in the anus).

REMEDIES
External
Make a poultice from boiled potatoes mashed with some butter. Sleep with the poultice in contact with the problem area throughout the night.

Internal

Symptoms include itching and painful defecation. Inject into the rectum with a syringe the following mixture:

- 50ml olive oil – cold pressed
- 50ml filtered lemon juice

If haemorrhoids bleed, insert 6 ice cubes into the rectal opening. Retain them there as long as you can bear it.

❋ Halitosis (bad breath)

BODY ORGANS
- stomach
- lungs
- thymus
- colon

SPINAL ADJUSTMENT
- cervical 1–4, thoracic 3–4–5–6–7–8, lumbar 1–5 and sacrum

This ailment is usually caused by an infection of the lower throat and/or the upper oesophagus and the mouth cavities. It is also a sign of inflammation of the sinuses or digestive problems.

FRESH JUICE RECIPE

Make 500ml from equal amounts of the following juices:
- carrot
- celery
- cucumber

Add a pinch of salt and black pepper and ½ teaspoon paprika. Drink undiluted. Chew mustard cress while drinking this juice.

In addition:

– Eat more alkaline-forming food.
– Practise breathing exercises.
– Chew some walnut bark into a pulp. Rub it on the gums and leave for 10 minutes. Gargle afterwards with lemon water.

❁ Hangovers

(See also Angry Liver)

REMEDIES

Champagne hangover
- orange juice
- 1 teaspoon coarse black pepper
- ice cubes

Wine hangover
- 1 tablespoon port
- 1 tablespoon brandy
- 1 cup hot water

General hangover
- juice of 2 lemons
- 1 teaspoon bicarbonate of soda
- cup hot water

Drink the mixture as it starts to froth.

Hair of the dog
- Drink more of the alcohol that caused the hangover in the first place.

❁ Hay fever

BODY ORGANS
- kidneys
- spleen

SPINAL ADJUSTMENT
- cervical 2–3–4

VAGUE SYMPTOMS
- sneezing
- itching nose
- red eyes

Hay fever can be caused by the use of drugs or an excessive amount of antibiotics during childhood. It may also be hereditary. If the hay fever is genetic you will need to work through your family history.

The majority of people who suffer from hay fever are allergic to pollen. As a consequence, when the pollen count increases they suffer a reaction. Certain foods – such as wheat, red meat, sugar and milk products – also tend to increase sufferers' susceptibility to hay fever. Use products which assist, such as honey, molasses and maple syrup instead of sugar; soya bean milk or unpasteurised goat's milk products instead of cow's milk products; maize, rice, barley, buckwheat and oats instead of wheat; fish and poultry instead of red meat.

The use of antihistamines is not advisable. They *lower* your resistance to the pollen thus increasing the need for antihistamine. Eventually you will require a complete cleanout of your entire system to re-establish your resistance.

Anticatarrhal foods are onions, garlic, chives, horseradish, mustard cress and watercress. Eat a balance of 70 per cent raw and 30 per cent cooked food. An ill-functioning colon or constipation is likely to increase the incidence of hay fever. I recommend the following drink.

FRESH JUICE RECIPE
Mix equal amounts of the following juices:
- celery
- carrot
- cooking apple

Take 450ml on an empty stomach, especially between May and August when the pollen count is highest.

For an immediate reaction when suffering, try a sniff of cold salt water. Mix 1 teaspoon of salt in a cup of filtered cold water. Sniff through the nose until the water emerges via the mouth. It may sting, but it will certainly help to clean the sinuses. You could also insert a drop of pure sesame oil into each nostril before going to bed. Chewing a honeycomb after removing the honey is another helpful remedy.

❋ Headaches

BODY ORGANS
• a headache can originate in any of the 12 body organs

SPINAL ADJUSTMENT
• entire cervical area

A headache is more a symptom than a disease, so do not suppress it. Instead, attempt to identify the cause. The main reason is usually insufficient elimination; when the liver is overworked, for instance, and cannot properly detoxify the system, a headache is one of the likely consequences. Headaches can also be symptomatic of nephritis, acitis, gastritis, hepatitis, iritis, meningitis or a tumour. The best prevention always is to care for yourself with love, rather than abuse your body as if it were a machine that requires no preventative maintenance or careful handling. When you have a headache, talk to your head. Ask it what it is attempting to tell you. Try to understand the signs, and listen carefully with your mind and your intuition.

If you require instant relief, use white willow bark tea instead of a headache pill. It contains salicylic acid, one of the ingredients in paracetamol, but here it is not synthetic or extracted.

If the headache is not a migraine, the following drink will help.

FRESH JUICE RECIPE
Mix equal amounts of the following juices to make 500ml:
• carrot
• spinach
• parsley
• raw beetroot
• cucumber
• cos lettuce

Add a pinch of salt and cumin powder and the juice of ½ lemon. Sip slowly, undiluted.

❋ Heart problems

SPINAL ADJUSTMENT
- cervical 1–2 and thoracic 2–3–4

VAGUE SYMPTOMS
- hearing your heartbeat when you rest the head on a pillow
- breathlessness
- fatigue

DISCOMFORT
- pain in the chest
- wooziness
- sudden syncope (fainting)

This remedy will help, provided that you are not suffering from a chronic heart disease.

FRESH JUICE RECIPE
Boil 1 tablespoon of hawthorn berries and ½ tablespoon lily of the valley in 500ml water until about 125ml is left. Mix with 500ml of equal amounts of the following juices:

- carrot
- spinach
- parsley
- cucumber

Add a pinch each of salt, black pepper and ginger. Drink 1–1½ litres daily.

❋ Herpes

BODY ORGANS
- lungs

SPINAL ADJUSTMENT
- genital herpes – lumbar 4–5
- oral herpes – cervical 1–2 and 5–6

There are 3 kinds of herpes:

- Herpes simplex – blisters on the lips during a cold

- Herpes zoster – within the nervous system
- Herpes genitalis – on the private parts

They all stem from the same kind of infection and occur when the body is too alkaline, even though we need a slightly alkaline body to avoid most diseases. The disadvantage of excessive alkalinity is a propensity towards ulcers, arthritis and herpes. There seems to be some truth in the idea that herpes is caused by the chicken pox vaccination, which is a weakened form of the virus.

With the onset of herpes on the lips or genitals, try eating broccoli steamed in a little water with soy sauce and lemon. Eat nothing else for 1 or 2 days until the attack has stopped. Thereafter concentrate on strengthening your immune system.

For breakfast eat 4 grilled oranges and nothing for 2 hours thereafter. Have a cold sitz bath for 3 minutes before bed.

❋ High blood pressure

BODY ORGANS
- lungs
- heart

SPINAL ADJUSTMENT
- thoracic 2–3–4

PSYCHOLOGICAL ASPECT
- holding the breath, pushing the heart to the extreme

VAGUE SYMPTOMS
- dizziness
- imbalance
- bloated feeling
- pounding in the temples

DISCOMFORT
- pain in the neck, headache
- indigestion
- dehydration
- lethargy
- fatigue

DIS-EASE
- high cholesterol
- clogged arteries
- stenosis (constriction of arteries)
- constipation
- craving for salt, or the use of too much salt

Boil 1 tablespoon of buckwheat in 500ml of water until 125ml is left. Buckwheat contains rutin, a substance which lowers the blood pressure by helping the capillaries to circulate blood more effectively. Remove the buckwheat and mix the remaining liquid with the following juice.

FRESH JUICE RECIPE
Make 375ml from equal amounts of the following juices:
- carrot
- cucumber
- spinach
- celery
- raw beetroot

Add a pinch each of salt, black pepper and ground roasted cumin seeds, and 1 teaspoon paprika. Eat ½ cos lettuce while drinking the juice. The outer leaves are more important than the inner.

Eat the boiled buckwheat during the day.

Prevention

Learn how to breathe out more effectively. Drink at least 2 litres of liquid a day. Avoid tinned and processed food. Eat raw foods instead. Add to your diet more bitter foods such as endives, bitter almonds, herbs, dandelion, gourds and sage tea.

❋ Hyperactivity

BODY ORGANS
- lungs
- kidneys
- heart

SPINAL ADJUSTMENT
- thoracic 9–10–12

Hyperactivity can be the result of renal, cardiac, psychosomatic or hepatic trouble.

REMEDIES

- Eliminate sugar from your diet.
- Drink cos lettuce soup.
- Eat a pinch of nutmeg to 'cool down' your nervous system (can also be used for hyperactive children and infants).
- Drink a cup of hot milk with honey and ¼ teaspoon of nutmeg before going to bed.

❋ Impotence

BODY ORGANS
- kidneys
- pelvis

EMOTIONAL ASPECTS
- fear and apprehension

REMEDY
- Masturbate (but do not ejaculate) twice a day for 28 days. After 28 days masturbate once a day for 56 days. Thereafter try sex with a partner, but avoid sex during the 84 days of masturbation.
- Eat cream cheese with celery and resist wheat and red meat.
- Improve pelvic circulation and have a cold sitz bath for 3 minutes before bed.
- Eat 100g of pumpkin seeds a day.
- Eat 10 oysters 3 times a week. If you are a vegetarian, eat more broccoli, pumpkin seeds and walnuts.

❋ Influenza

BODY ORGANS
- immune system
- lungs
- colon

SPINAL ADJUSTMENT
- cervical

FIRST SYMPTOMS
- sneezing
- sore throat
- exhaustion
- fever
- itching nose, throat, eyes

REMEDIES
- Drink onion soup made from 200g of red onion with paprika, black pepper and tabasco. Make it very hot.
- Eat grilled oranges for breakfast for 7 days.
- Chew 20 peppercorns followed by hot water.
- Inhale the vapours from 10 drops of eucalyptus oil, 10 drops of tea tree oil and 10 drops of Olbas oil mixed in a basin of hot water.
- Take 1,000g vitamin C effervescent tablets every 2 hours for 48 hours.
- Cold sponge down the entire length of the spine before bed.

FRESH JUICE RECIPE
Make 375ml from equal amounts of the following juices:
- carrot
- celery
- cucumber
- spinach
- lemon (with pith)
- grapefruit (with pith)

Dilute with 125ml of slightly cooled boiled water. Drink 2–3 litres a day.

✳ Insomnia

Insomnia often afflicts busy people who never have enough time. They are often extroverts who are unable to switch off their minds.

BODY ORGANS
- lungs
- heart
- central nervous system
- kidneys
- stomach

SPINAL ADJUSTMENT
- upper cervical

EMOTIONS
- apprehension
- lack of joy

VAGUE SYMPTOMS
- sleeplessness – physical, emotional and mental disturbance
- restlessness and spiritual lethargy
- not feeling fresh in the morning
- waking up feeling unwell and worried
- heavy sweating while asleep
- acute awareness of passing time

DISEASE
- pain
- an acute disease
- brain tumour

You may be unable to sleep for many reasons – perhaps you are over-tired or your digestive system is too full with food, or you may have worries and concerns. Regardless of the cause, sleeping pills will not help in the long term. Their effect is minimized as the body gets used to them.

My initial suggestion is that you reduce the volume of stale air in your lungs. Lie down and breathe in and out 50 times, forcing the air out. Concentrate on your out-breaths and let your in-breaths take care of themselves. This exercise should help you to relax. It can also be helpful to learn to sigh, and to stretch as many of your muscles as possible before going to bed. Thirdly, I suggest having a hot and cold shower last thing at night.

My fourth suggestion is dietary. Finely chop some cos lettuce, about 6–8 outer leaves and the stem. Sauté in oil with 2 sticks of cinnamon, 2 cloves and, if you want to add taste, ½ red onion, finely chopped. Add a pinch of salt and black pepper, and a few drops of lemon. Eat about half an hour before going to bed – and then do the breathing exercise.

Or try these drinks; they may help you to relax.

FRESH JUICE RECIPE
Mix together equal amounts of the following juices:
- cos lettuce
- carrot
- spinach
- celery

Drink 1½–2 litres a day, undiluted.

Before going to bed prepare a drink consisting of the juice of 1 lemon, 1 teaspoon of honey and ¼ teaspoon of nutmeg powder in a cup of boiled hot water.

Serotinin
Serotonin is a neural transmitter which calms the system. A basic source of serotonin is tryptophan, an amino acid found in foods such as sweet biscuits and sweet crackers. Eat more of these sweet foods and chew them slowly. This will liberate the sugar to produce serotonin in your brain and relax the body. Reduce the amount of protein in your food and eat fewer milk products to lower your acid level. The combination of serotonin and a lower acid level will act as a powerful soporific.

❄ Kidney stones

SPINAL ADJUSTMENT
- lumbar 2–3–4

VAGUE SYMPTOMS
- lower backache

- strong smelling urine, from proteins and other deposits
- thirst

DISCOMFORT
- spasm in the lower back
- change in perspiration
- acute pains in the lower back and kidney area
- brittle hair and nails
- fever
- desire for salt
- lethargy

Food enters the bloodstream through hepatic veins and the villi in the small intestines. The blood is filtered in the liver before circulating through the lungs, where the blood is infused with oxygen before moving on to the heart. The blood then leaves the heart via the aorta to the kidneys where it is purified. The liver filters out toxins of food, alcohol and bacteria, and stores glycogen to convert into glucose when needed. The kidneys ensure hormonal balance (sexual hormones), maintain electrolyte balance (mineral balance), and control the blood sugar via the adrenal glands.

Kidney stones form when the kidneys fail to filter properly or as a result of nephritis.

REMEDIES
Take 60g of fresh vine leaves and make tea from them. Drink 3 cups daily. This should dissolve the stones. It can be a most painful experience when the stones emerge. To release the tension, hold a ginger compress (see Appendix B) around the painful area, which is right and left of the spine at lumbar 1 and thoracic 12.

If vine leaves are not available, make 6 litres of watermelon juice. (Use the entire watermelon, including the green parts, but not the skin or the seeds.) Boil down to 3 litres and drink all of it in 1 day.

Have a cold sitz bath before going to bed.

On rising, take the juice of 1 lemon in a cup of hot water.

FRESH JUICE RECIPE
Boil 1 tablespoon dandelion (from the herbalist) in 500ml of water until 125ml is left. Combine equal amounts of the following juices to make 375ml:

- carrot
- spinach
- celery
- cucumber
- grape

Mix the juice with the reduced dandelion water and the juice of a lemon. Drink 1½ litres a day.

❋ Lethargy

Biologically, the cause of lethargy is lack of haemoglobin. It can be one of the after-effects of an infection that has left the body weakened. Lethargy can also be the result of a psychosomatic disease.

BODY ORGANS
- lungs

SPINAL ADJUSTMENT
- entire cervical area

EMOTION
- apprehension

VAGUE SYMPTOMS
- shallow breathing
- sluggish circulation
- indecision
- lack of energy

DIS-EASE:
- chronic dormant infection

The key to increasing your energy level is to improve your breathing. Try the following.

- Breathe deeply and sigh. Force out-breaths to completely clean out the lungs. The best time for breathing exercises is first thing in the morning.
- Practise Tantric exercises.

❋ Liver problems

VAGUE SYMPTOMS
• bitter taste in the mouth

DISCOMFORT
• constipation
• itching
• pressure in the solar plexus area
• no appetite
• lack of energy
• oversensitivity to fatty foods

The liver is our second largest organ (the skin is the largest), and is the only organ that can regenerate itself. Like a lizard which has had its tail cut off, the liver can recreate part of itself. But once the liver has cirrhosis and the cells have become fibrous, it loses its regenerative capability. However, given sufficient time, even fibrous liver cells, such as occur in hepatitis, can be repaired.

The main functions of the liver are: the storage and metabolism of proteins, carbohydrates and glucose; the detoxification of foreign invaders and toxins that the body itself produces; the production of bile; the provision of iron for blood cell production; the storage of blood and glycogen; and the purification of bacterial invaders. The liver also divides nutritional sources into deposits, material for bile, and waste products. It resolves the problems of putrefaction when food becomes fermented and stale.

The liver is therefore a most important organ. Sometimes it can become inflamed. Any monofast consisting of a single fruit or vegetable, or their juices, will bring relief to an infected liver. Grapes and plums provide the best relief.

Quite remarkably, the liver is 1½ degrees higher in temperature than the rest of the body. It also helps maintain body temperature. The liver depends upon the kidneys to filter minerals. When the kidneys fail to perform this function properly the work-load of the liver is doubled. (See the entry for kidney stones.)

The liver can also be poisoned by the colon if elimination is incomplete. It is therefore important to ensure that the bowels function efficiently.

Drink the following juice when discomfort occurs, in order to maintain the functions of the liver.

FRESH JUICE RECIPE
Take 1 tablespoon of dandelion with roots (from a herbalist) and boil in 500ml of water until 125ml remains. Add 375ml of equal amounts of the following juices:

- carrot
- raw beetroot
- parsley
- radishes (with leaves)

Drink 1½ litres a day.

Avoid fatty foods and alcohol.

❋ Menopausal problems

BODY ORGANS
- uterus
- kidneys
- ovaries
- spleen

SPINAL ADJUSTMENT
- lower thoracic and upper lumbar

Hormonal balance can be achieved with the help of natural remedies. Once this is achieved, the body is better equipped to take care of itself. Hormone tablets are unnecessary if you think of the menopause in terms of freedom rather than bondage.

REMEDIES

- Have a cold sitz bath for 3 minutes every night before going to bed (see Appendix B). Rub yourself dry with a warm towel.
- Have foot massages, concentrating on the reflex points for the kidneys and spleen.
- Eat more broccoli, cos lettuce and pumpkin seeds.

– Seek further advice on the use and benefits of vitamins and herbs from a herbalist or healing practitioner.

✳ Migraine

For a better understanding see also Headaches.

PRACTICAL TIPS
– Put your head under cold water for 30 seconds to 1 minute, then rub thoroughly with a towel.
– Go for a walk in the fresh air and free your spirit by shouting to the universe (whatever comes to mind) provided you can handle the reactions of more conventional onlookers!
– Make a cos lettuce soup (see recipe in Appendix C). Add nutmeg.
– Take one 250mg tablet of B6 before going to bed (women only).

FRESH JUICE RECIPE
Make 375ml from equal amounts of the following juices:
• carrot
• spinach
• celery
• parsley

Dilute with 125ml boiled water that has slightly cooled. Add ¼ teaspoon nutmeg powder, a pinch each of salt, black pepper and cardamom powder.

✳ Mouth blisters

BODY ORGANS
• colon
• stomach

SPINAL ADJUSTMENT
• thoracic 6–7–8

REMEDIES
Chew some walnut bark and clean the affected area. Make sure you eat a blend of foods that is not too acidic.

❋ Nails – brittle

BODY ORGAN
- kidneys

EMOTIONAL ASPECT
- fear

REMEDIES
- Find out what the fear is about and work on it.
- Drink more water (bottled or filtered).
- Eat watermelon, nori (seaweed), 20 almonds a day, fresh fish.
- Avoid wheat and sugar.

❋ Nerve problems

BODY ORGANS
- central nervous system

SPINAL ADJUSTMENT
- cervical 3–4–5 and thoracic 4–5–6

VAGUE SYMPTOMS
- sleeplessness
- nail biting
- fidgeting
- depression

It is important to exercise regularly, and to practise deep breathing, relaxation, meditation and centring. Most nervous symptoms tend to be psychological in origin.

FRESH JUICE RECIPE
Combine equal amounts of the following juices:
- carrot
- celery
- spinach
- cucumber

Drink 2–3 litres a day, undiluted.

❈ Ovarian tumour

BODY ORGANS
• uterus

SPINAL ADJUSTMENT
• entire lumbar area

Ovarian tumours can be quite large, the size of a grapefruit in some cases. It is a strange coincidence in my opinion that a number of women with ovarian tumours have a strong desire to conceive. Perhaps in these cases the body responds by producing a phantom baby. If you are in this situation, may I suggest that you find ways to legitimately hug and cuddle children so that your motherly instincts are fulfilled.

If you suspect an ovarian tumour, always seek professional advice. A common remedy that may help is to take a cold sitz bath for 3 minutes every night before going to bed. Rub yourself thoroughly dry to increase the circulation to all the pelvic organs.

❈ Palpitations of the heart

BODY ORGANS
• heart
• small intestines
• kidneys

EMOTIONS
• anxiety

SPINAL ADJUSTMENT
• thoracic 3–5

Palpitations can be the result of:
• heart disease
• inflammation of the stomach
• hyperadrenaline
• constant worry

REMEDIES
- nutmeg powder (to stimulate the psyche)
- pumpkin seeds
- cos lettuce salad
- garlic (to bring down the blood pressure)

Learn to breathe deeply. Find ways to deal with anxiety.

✳ Pelvic trouble

BODY ORGANS
- kidneys
- large intestines

EMOTIONS
- fear
- uptightness

SPINAL ADJUSTMENT
- lower lumbar

VAGUE SYMPTOMS
- bad circulation
- cold feet, cold bottom
- sweaty soles of the feet
- cramps in the calf muscles

DISCOMFORT
- prostate or uterine problems
- impotence or frigidity
- dismenorrhoea or amenorrhoea

DIS-EASE
- lower back pain
- haemorrhoids caused by constipation
- infertility
- groin pain
- lymphatic disorders

DISEASE
- prostatitis
- ovarian cyst
- uterine cancer

Take a cold sitz bath for 3 minutes before going to bed every night. Perform a cleansing diet.

❋ Pregnancy problems

GENERAL ADVICE
- Avoid negative thoughts.
- Do not get constipated.
- Do not indulge in drugs.
- Perform deep breathing exercises for at least half an hour a day.
- Do not overload your system with heavy protein meals (use the ratio 2 protein/2 starch/6 mineral).

FRESH JUICE RECIPE
Boil 1 tablespoon raspberries and their leaves in 500ml of water until 125ml is left. Combine equal amounts of the following juices to make 375ml:

- carrot
- celery
- raw beetroot
- cucumber
- fresh coconut
- cooking apple

Mix the juice with the raspberry water. Add a pinch each of salt, black pepper, clove powder and ground roasted black jeera or cumin seeds. Drink 1 litre a day. Eat 1 large orange with each cup.

❃ Sexual problems

BODY ORGANS
- kidneys (men)
- uterus and ovaries (women)

SPINAL ADJUSTMENT
- entire lumbar area and sacrum

VAGUE SYMPTOMS
- dribbling

DISCOMFORT
- polyuria

DIS-EASE
- impotence, inability to ejaculate
- vaginal dryness, lack of desire

For 14 days eat the following dish with your evening meal. Mix together 250g of assorted green vegetables. Shred and warm in a pan, adding 100g of fresh fish roes.

Try sex again on the 14th day.

❃ Shingles

BODY ORGANS
- lungs
- colon
- immune system

SPINAL ADJUSTMENT
- cervical, thoracic and lumbar – depending on where the lesion occurs

Shingles is a rash of herpes zoster. It follows the neural pathways.

For some relief from the itching pain, make the following preparation:
- 50 per cent extract of hamamelis
- 50 per cent spirits of camphor

Mix and apply to affected areas.

Strengthen the immune system and laugh for 5 minutes a day.

❋ Sinusitis

BODY ORGANS
- colon
- lungs

EMOTION
- apprehension

SPINAL ADJUSTMENT
- entire cervical area

Sinusitis is an inflammation of the facial sinuses. Sufferers are mostly people who do not eliminate completely, who have bad eating habits, or who do not breathe properly and are congested much of the time. Allergies are usually genetic. If, for instance, you have a family history of, or a particular propensity to asthma or diabetes, you need to be aware of the possibility of your own allergic disposition.

The foods which cause the strongest reactions are wheat, sugar, milk, red meat, tinned food, over-processed and junk foods. Microwave cooking is another likely cause. Avoid microwave food for at least 3–6 months to recover from the effects. Try not to buy pre-cooked foods. Eat more fresh vegetables, especially root vegetables. Anticatarrhal foods include chives, garlic, red onions (not white), mustard cress, horseradish, ordinary mustard, endives. Endives are very rich and bitter, but highly anticatarrhal.

Eat more grains, lentils and legumes instead of animal protein. If you do eat protein, avoid over-processed foods such as sausages and pies. If you must eat protein, try not to mix it with carbohydrates. For example, instead of a ham sandwich, eat a sandwich with banana or tomato or salad. Although not 'complete proteins' they will provide you with essential amino acids. Food combining is most important. If you do eat food such as fried bread or a traditional English breakfast, try to have it with a side salad. This will reduce the risk of inflammation.

INSTANT RELIEF

To reduce an acute attack, put 20 drops of eucalyptus oil or Olbas oil or camphor oil into a basin of boiling water. Put a towel over your head and inhale. Keep your eyes closed to avoid stinging. This will relieve the inflammation of the sinuses.

If you are brave, learn to sniff water through your nose until it comes out of your mouth. This exercise will keep your nasal passages clean. Before going to bed, a drop of sesame oil in each nostril will help to reduce inflammation.

FRESH JUICE RECIPE

Combine equal amounts of the following juices:

- carrot
- spinach
- cucumber
- lemon

Add ¼ teaspoon of mustard powder, ¼ teaspoon of nutmeg powder, a pinch each of salt, black pepper and ground roasted cumin seeds. Drink 1–1½ litres a day, undiluted.

❋ Skin problems

Irritation

BODY ORGANS

- lungs
- colon

SPINAL ADJUSTMENT

- upper thoracic

DISCOMFORT

- itching
- redness

REMEDIES

– Focus on breathing out to expel the air and allow in-breathing to take care of itself.

- Rub cider vinegar all over the body, leave for 10 minutes then have a shower.
- Drink onion soup made from 200g red onions every day.
- Have ½ cos lettuce a day (raw or cooked).
- Eat as much raw food as you can.

FRESH JUICE RECIPE
Prepare 750ml from equal amounts of the following juices:
- celery
- carrot
- cucumber

Drink half for breakfast and the remaining half later in the day.

Dry skin

Mix together the following:
- 50ml olive oil
- 10 drops rose oil
- 10 drops sandalwood oil
- 10 drops rosemary oil

Rub onto your body and leave for 20 minutes before going to bed.

Focus on emptying the lungs and expelling all the stale air.

Hard skin

Get rid of hard skin on the feet by rubbing it off with a pumice stone. Then apply cider vinegar every day for 3 months.

❋ Sore throats

BODY ORGANS
- lungs
- colon

EMOTION
- stress – the system is depleted by depression

SPINAL ADJUSTMENT
- lower cervical 7–6–5, upper thoracic 3–5

A sore throat can be the result of over-use or an infection. An inability to swallow suggests inflammation.

REMEDIES
– To soothe the inflammation, use glycerine mixed with bicarbonate of soda. Attach cotton wool securely to the end of a long clean stick, dip it in the mixture and apply it *very carefully* to the uvula at the back of your throat, or have a friend perform this action for you.
– If your condition is chronic and glycerine or bicarbonate of soda are not immediately available, you can use sage. Chew some fresh green rather than red sage. Swallow it once it is thoroughly chewed. It will help to soothe your throat. If you do not have fresh sage, boil 1 teaspoon of dried sage in a cup of water. Filter and use the water to gargle gently.

Inflamed tonsils

A sore throat can also be caused by inflamed tonsils. The tonsils are the body's soldiers – their role is to prevent infection from entering the body. When they become infected, it is a sign that they are protecting you. It will nevertheless help to address the inflammation. Gargle with bicarbonate of soda. Add some lemon and 1 teaspoon of honey if your tonsils are particularly sore, but *swallow* the mixture after gargling, unlike other gargle solutions which are spat out.

❋ Sweaty hands

BODY ORGANS
- lungs
- colon

EMOTIONAL ASPECT
- apprehension – being unsure of yourself

Release the energy meridian of the lungs and colon. Perform 50 swings with your arms, clockwise and anticlockwise. Have hot and cold showers on the spine daily.

❋ Thrush

BODY ORGANS
- stomach
- spleen

SYMPTOMS
- in the mouth – painful white coating on the tongue
- on the genitals – redness, itching, a creamy discharge

Thrush can occur in the mouth or on the genitals. It can sometimes be an immune deficiency reaction (the immune system reacting in a defective manner) following the intake of antibiotics.

If thrush moves internally from the tongue to the large intestine, you may find the following prescription useful. (Thuja is available from healthfood stores or homoeopathic chemists.)
- Take 1 dose of thuja 200D every night for 7 days, 1 dose of thuja CM on the 8th day, and 1 dose of thuja 6D each morning and evening for 7 days thereafter.

REMEDIES
- Take a cold sitz bath for 3 minutes before going to bed.
- Exclude all sugar from your diet.
- Take 1 tablet of Coenzyme Q10 a day.
- Drink a fresh fruit juice and a revitalization juice (see page 62) on alternate days.

❋ Tonsillitis

BODY ORGANS
- immune system
- lungs
- colon

SPINAL ADJUSTMENT
- upper cervical

VAGUE SYMPTOMS
- breathing difficulties
- swallowing difficulties

DISCOMFORT
- fever
- swollen neck and glands
- constipation
- high fever and diarrhoea

Try fasting, eating only grilled oranges for 3 days, or any other fruit (one kind of fruit only). Eat as much of the chosen fruit as you wish.

FRESH JUICE RECIPE
Mix together equal amounts of the following juices:
- carrot
- celery
- pineapple
- orange
- lemon

Add a pinch of salt, black pepper and mustard powder. Drink 1½ litres of undiluted juice a day.

Gargle with sage tea. Afterwards dust the tonsils with dry turmeric powder. Use a swab as described in the Sore Throats entry. Do this 3–4 times a day.

❋ Urticaria (nettle rash, hives, wheals)

BODY ORGANS
- lungs
- colon
- kidneys
- liver

SPINAL ADJUSTMENT
- upper cervical

SYMPTOMS
- itching and a rash
- raised red blotches or wheals

Urticaria is caused by a lack of calcium, sodium or magnesium, or if minerals are not properly utilized. Skin respiration is then blocked.

FRESH JUICE RECIPE

Mix together equal amounts of the following juices:

- carrot
- raw beetroot
- spinach
- celery
- cooking apple

Add a pinch of salt, ¼ teaspoon fenugreek powder and ¼ teaspoon basil leaves. Drink 1 litre a day, undiluted. Eat 20 unpeeled almonds (soaked overnight) while drinking the juice.

❋ Varicose veins (varicosis)

BODY ORGANS

- heart
- lungs
- liver

SPINAL ADJUSTMENT

- lower lumbar

VAGUE SYMPTOMS

- fatigue

Varicose veins are hereditary. If either of your parents had varicose veins, there is a reasonable chance that you will also be a sufferer. Treatment can but slow down the onset of this degenerative process.

Prevention

- Do not allow yourself to become constipated. Ensure that you have 1–2 bowel movements a day.
- Do not sit cross-legged. This position tends to block the blood flow.
- Eat at least 100g of uncooked beetroot a day.
- Drink buckwheat water with juniper berries or 2–3 cups of buckwheat leaf tea a day.
- Have a cold sitz bath for 3 minutes before going to bed. Dry yourself vigorously with a warm towel.

FRESH JUICE RECIPE
Mix together equal amounts of the following juices to make 375ml:
- celery
- spinach
- watercress
- mustard cress
- green pepper

Add 125ml of buckwheat water.

❋ Verrucas and warts

BODY ORGANS
- lungs
- colon

SPINAL ADJUSTMENT
- upper thoracic – to improve the operation of the lungs

Verrucas

A verruca is a form of skin irritation. It is a single root fungus which usually attacks the fingers and toes. It occurs when the outer skin is too alkaline and not entirely clean. Lowered resistance increases the likelihood of infection.

The first way to deal with a verruca is to make the skin acidic by having Epsom salts baths. Then clean the entire area with cider vinegar. Once a verruca begins to spread it is difficult to contain and becomes most painful.

REMEDIES
The simplest and most effective remedy is baked onion. Bake a small onion, remove the centre and put the onion on the verruca. Allow the onion to foment to your tolerance limit. Leave it in place overnight. Repeat each day for 3–5 days.

Another good remedy is tincture of thuja, which you can buy from any healthfood store or homoeopathic chemist. Apply before going to bed. It will help to increase the acidity of the skin. Remember that for a healthy balance the skin needs to be acidic and the inside of the body slightly alkaline.

Verrucas on the feet are particularly difficult to deal with because pressure is applied to them constantly. The only solution is to have a chiropodist remove the root. Once this has been done, consider the following recommendations.

Prevention

– Change your socks twice a day.
– Change your shoes frequently (wear the same pair only once every 4 days).
– Do not wear rubber-soled shoes (they prevent the feet from breathing adequately).

REMEDY
Mash ripe banana into a pulp, apply to the verruca and cover with a plaster. Alternatively, use unheated liquid honey. It is important to keep the plaster on for 48 hours, so do not allow the foot to get wet when you shower or bath during this period. After removing the plaster, wash the verruca with cider vinegar.

Warts

Apply your saliva to the warts as many times as possible during the day. You can also put crushed garlic on them, held in place with a plaster. Alternatively, use the juice from a fresh mango or papaya.

FRESH JUICE RECIPE
Boil 1 tablespoon of dandelion roots and leaf (from a herbalist) in 500ml water and reduce to 125ml. Add to 375ml of equal amounts of the following juices:

- watercress
- mustard cress
- cos lettuce
- spinach
- celery

Add a pinch each of salt, black pepper and mustard powder and 1 teaspoon of paprika.

REMEDY
Apply thuja tincture 4 times a day until the wart has vanished.

❋ Vomiting

BODY ORGANS
- stomach
- pancreas
- liver
- spleen

Vomiting can occur suddenly. It can happen for a number of reasons – you have eaten stale food; you have some kind of disease; some food has become lodged; you are suffering from food poisoning. Vomiting is the body's reaction to food that it cannot handle. It is nature's way of eliminating a substance that is injurious to the body, so do not attempt to stop the process. Afterwards, try to further clear the system by drinking plenty of water. This will also have the effect of diluting the cause of the illness.

AFTERCARE
Boil 1 teaspoon of fennel and 1 teaspoon of dill seeds in 3 cups of water. Ensure that the container is enamel or stainless steel and not aluminium. Boil it until 1 cup is left. Filter it and take 1 tablespoon every 2 hours (1 teaspoon for children).

The moment that your body is able to retain something stronger, try a tea that will calm the system such as ginger, camomile, mint or any herbal tea. Boil 1 tablespoon of grated fresh ginger in 3 cups of water until 1 cup remains. Filter the water and drink it slowly. Then eat more alkaline foods, like yoghurt with banana, which will further soothe your system.

It is important to bring up the entire stomach contents, and not to worry about the vomiting – unless you are suffering from bulimia, ulcers or hiatus hernia. If the vomiting continues for longer than 24 hours, seek professional help.

❋ Wrinkles

BODY ORGANS
- lungs
- spleen
- colon
- kidneys

SPINAL ADJUSTMENT
- the cervical area – to increase the circulation in the neck

Try cucumber slices packed around the eyes. It is an astringent and can be used effectively against wrinkles.

Cut down your intake of milk, sugar and other foods to which you might have an allergic reaction. Eat less meat. Apply sesame oil to your face instead of face cream.

People who relive and regret the past are more prone to wrinkles, as are those who blame themselves and other people for their life circumstances.

Try to have more sex – and decide to be happy. Remember, pain creates wrinkles, laughter removes them.

Finally, some general advice on Antibiotics and Slimming.

❋ Antibiotics

The body has an inbuilt intelligence which enables it to generate its own antibiotics in response to illness. The use of artificial antibiotics inhibits the body's ability to marshal its own defences. Consequently, the dosage of these antibiotics needs to be constantly increased to maintain their effectiveness, thereby destroying some of the intestinal flora.

It is important after using artificial antibiotics to restore the intestinal flora. *Bifidus* bacteria which are intestine-friendly are found in yoghurt. Bananas are also good for the intestines and nourish the *bifidus* bacteria.

FOR BREAKFAST

Mash together 2 overripe bananas with 125g bioyoghurt. *Do not* add other fruit, nuts or honey as they will destroy the vitality of the enzymes whose strength you are attempting to enhance. Continue this breakfast remedy for at least 1 month.

❋ Slimming

BODY ORGANS
- kidneys
- spleen
- liver

SPINAL ADJUSTMENT
- lower thoracic and upper lumbar

EMOTIONAL ASPECT
- all emotions suppressed

PSYCHOLOGICAL ASPECTS
- self-hate
- self-destruction

A certain amount of body fat is essential for our wellbeing. Most people who put on weight have a sweet tooth and eat an excessive amount of carbohydrates. If you want to slim, you may find the following notes useful.

Learn to eat only when you are hungry and stop eating before you feel bloated. Do not eat just to feel full. Eat slowly and chew your food thoroughly. Eat more proteins and minerals, and fewer carbohydrates.

There are 8 different tastes available to us (see Appendix A). Most of us, however, are content with only 3 – salty, sweet and sour. If we shift our food balance to include the other 5 – bitter, pungent, astringent, putrid, and hot – our body will be able to eliminate waste more completely. The less frequently used tastes will increase our metabolic rate and enable the body to digest food more thoroughly. As a consequence, less fat will be dumped and stored in the body.

It is also important for the skin to remain acidic. Have lots of hot baths as this will ensure that the pores remain open. Take care not to get constipated. Take lots of exercise, including long walks. Remember, singing is also a very effective exercise.

Finally, steer well clear of slimming pills and remember to eat only when you are hungry.

PART III

<u>FOOD AS MEDICINE</u>

CHAPTER 11

The Healing Qualities of Natural Food Sources

❋ Alfalfa

– contains all the essential minerals; rich in zinc and iron; makes the body less acidic

TASTE bitter
ELEMENT fire

Nutritional value
- one of the richest, known sources of organic salts – especially potassium, iron, zinc, magnesium, phosphorus and calcium – and of all plants the richest in chlorophyll (2 per cent)
- contains vitamins A, B, D, E and G, some vitamin C, and the blood-clotting vitamin K
- rich in lysine and tryptophane (essential amino acids)
- contains sterole, which produces sex hormones

Did you know?
The alkalizing effect of alfalfa is outstanding: 100g contains 130.42 units of alkali-forming elements – more than lettuce or spinach but less than seaweed (about 180 units). (See the alkaline diet, p. 41.) The content of protein in alfalfa is between 1 and 1½ times greater than that in wheat or corn.

Natural therapeutic effects
- laxative, digestive, diuretic, tonic

Beneficial in the treatment of
- dropsy
- inflammation of kidneys
- immune system weaknesses
- hard arteries
- anaemia – the high amount of iron makes it a good therapeutic for anaemia and dental decay
- all arthritic diseases – because of its high alkalizing effect

❋ Almonds

– recalcifier; more nutritious than cow's milk and 100 per cent superior

TASTE bitter or sweet
ELEMENT earth

Nutritional value
- rich in calcium, manganese, phosphorus, potassium, magnesium, iron, vitamin A
- contain 59 per cent fat, 21 per cent protein

Did you know?
75–100g of almonds eaten daily will supply you with all the protein your body requires. It can be used as a substitute for meat or milk. Almond milk (see recipe below) is highly nutritious, but the skin has irritating properties and should not be eaten. It is best to soak almonds overnight and blanch and peel them the next morning. Almonds do not decay if they are kept dry, because they contain no putrefactive bacteria. Their emollient properties allay irritation of the skin and alleviate swelling and pain. This makes them an acceptable ingredient in cosmetics.

Beneficial in the treatment of
- colon and bowel problems – can lessen the putrefactive effect of many foods

- asthma and skin diseases, which can be provoked by cow's milk, eggs and meat – act as an antidote
- diabetes
- rickets
- nephritis
- typhoid fever
- diarrhoea
- malnutrition
- secondary anaemia
- hyperacidity
- disturbances of gastric motility and secretion
- uric acid diathesis
- kidney disease
- peritonic irritation
- weak muscles, nerves and brain

Almonds mixed with figs are an instant laxative if chewed throroughly.

Sweet almonds

Natural therapeutic effects
- antiputrefactive, tonic

They are beneficial in the treatment of osteoporosis and when extra calcium is needed, for example:
- during the menopause
- for children during growth
- to heal a broken bone

ALMOND MILK RECIPE
225g of sweet almonds will produce between 1 and 1½ litres of milk. Soak overnight, blanch, peel and blend into a paste and add water. The liquid will then have the same structure as milk and can be processed into curd or butter.

Bitter almonds

– strengthen the immune system; anticancerous; blood-purifier

Natural therapeutic effect
- sedative

They contain cyanide, which is what gives them their bitter taste. They are useful in the treatment of cancer because they inhibit the growth of random cells. Bitter almonds also have calming properties.

Almond oil

Almond oil is used for earache, especially when it has been brought on by a cold, draughts or rheumatism. Put 7–8 drops into one ear and the next day the same quantity into the other ear. Syringe each ear the day after inserting the drops.

Tumours that generate great heat (inflammation) should be rubbed softly with almond oil. It will have a cooling effect.

For lung inflammation take 1 teaspoon 3–4 times a day.

❋ Aniseed

– relieves flatulence; helps digestion

TASTE pungent and sweet
ELEMENT metal

Nutritional value
• carminative (relieves flatulence), stomachic, antispasmodic

Did you know?
Aniseed can be used to balance the effect of coffee. (See the recipe for coffee in Appendix C.)

Natural therapeutic effects
• diuretic, carminative, antispasmodic, digestive, expectorant, stimulant, stomachic, tonic

Beneficial in the treatment of
• bad digestion
• flatulence
• cramps
• colic
• nausea

❋ Apples

– blood-purifier; cooked apples are good for diarrhoea

TASTE sour
ELEMENT wood

Nutritional value
- rich in potassium, sodium, vitamin A, vitamin G
- abundant source of vitamins A, C, B1, niacine and panthothenic acid
- 1 litre of apple juice contains 3–4½g of minerals

Did you know?
The large amount of phosphorus contained in apples makes them valuable as brain and nerve food, especially in cases of nervous exhaustion. They help 'brain' workers to stay clear and relaxed. Vitamin C is found in the skin of the apple.

Apples and pears are the only fruit that reveal a pentagonal shape in the centre when cut open. Each star contains a seed which is rich in arsen, a blood purifier. When you chew the seeds they will taste like almonds. Eating them will aid your digestion of the apple. But *be careful*. A cupful of apple seeds is sufficient to cause death.

Sour cooking apples are a useful appetiser. Cut them into slices and add salt and pepper. As an hors-d'oeuvre they will generate saliva and stimulate your appetite.

The most nutritious apples are custard apples, which are very sweet and filling.

Natural therapeutic effect
- cleansing

Beneficial in the treatment of
- sluggish bowels – cooking apples contain pectin, which absorbs excess water in the intestines and forms a solution that stimulates the bowels. Diarrhoea after eating apples is a sign that the cleansing process has started. **Caution:** a raw apple diet will usually produce intestinal catarrh and dysentery.
- burns – if you do not have a potato, tofu or honey and you suffer a first-degree burn, cut a slice of apple and put it on the burn immediately.

Hold it in place with a plaster. The apple will prevent the burn from blistering.
- arthritic complaints and gout – apples are rich in citric and malic acid, which have the ability to neutralize excessive acidity in the blood. Apple skins are useful to minimize an excessive level of uric acid in the blood.
- kidney disorders and skin afflictions – the large amounts of potassium salts in apples have a diuretic effect.
- kidney stones – cider is recommended as a preventative.
- hypertension – apples reduce the sodium content in the tissues, thereby reducing hypertension and blood pressure.
- high blood cholesterol – apples minimize the appetite and thereby lower blood cholesterol.
- inebriation, dyspepsia, weak digestion, headaches, biliousness, autointoxication and constipation.

❉ Apricots

– prevent constipation; improve memory

TASTE sweet
ELEMENT earth

Nutritional value
- rich in potassium, sodium, magnesium, iron

Did you know?
Dried apricots are a rich healing source, especially Hunza apricots from India which contain a high concentration of beta carotene. The cleansing effect on the colon will help to improve breathing, which will in turn strengthen the lungs. More oxygen means more brain activity and improved memory. This is of particular relevance for older people.

Natural therapeutic effects
- cathartic, tonic

Beneficial in the treatment of
- constipation – dried apricots are a most effective laxative

- cancer – especially of the skin, lungs and larynx. As a supplement to cancer treatment, eat 20 Hunza apricots for breakfast. They are a good source of vitamin B17. Soak them overnight and eat the next morning. Remember to open the kernel and eat the nut inside (see below).

❈ Apricot kernels

– anticancerous, blood purifier

TASTE bitter
ELEMENT fire

Nutritional value
- rich in cyanide (amygdalin) which, please note, is *poisonous* – take care particularly where children are involved

Did you know?
The nut of the apricot is rich in protein and fat and is made up of between 40 and 45 per cent oil. This oil is almost identical in its make-up to almond oil.

Beneficial in the treatment of
- cancer – can be used to control cancerous growths

Caution
Eat only a very small amount.

❈ Arnica

– for wounds, bruises, shock and post-trauma

TASTE bitter
ELEMENT fire

Did you know?
Arnica can be used for shock, including post-operative shock. Arnica should be used internally in the form of homoeopathic drops or pills, although it can also be applied externally to the skin.

Natural therapeutic effects
- diaphoretic, diuretic, emollient, expectorant, stimulant, vulnerary

Beneficial in the treatment of
- shock
- bruises
- swellings
- wounds

✽ Artichokes (globe, not Jerusalem)

– kidney tonic; dissolve kidney stones

TASTE bitter
ELEMENT fire

Nutritional value
- rich in potassium, calcium, iron and sulphur
- contain cynarin

Did you know?
The artichoke is an aphrodisiac and promotes seminal fluid. Whilst there is no cure for baldness, artichoke leaves, boiled and rubbed into the scalp, may retard hair loss.

 HAIR

Natural therapeutic effects
- cholagogic, diuretic

Beneficial in the treatment of
- kidney complaints
- jaundice
- dyspepsia
- liver insufficiency
- chronic albuminuria (proteins in the urine) *see also 146 + 204*
- arteriosclerosis (hardening of the arteries)
- high blood cholesterol

Caution
Never mix artichokes with asparagus.

❈ Asparagus

– kidney tonic; expels uric acid from the system

TASTE sweet
ELEMENT earth

Nutritional value
- rich in potassium

Natural therapeutic effects
- aperient (laxative), diaphoretic, diuretic

Beneficial in the treatment of
- rheumatic complaints
- multiple sclerosis
- cardiac dropsy
- chronic gout

Caution
Avoid if you have an advanced disease of the kidneys. Asparagus increases urine production and cellular activity in the kidneys.

Never mix asparagus with artichokes.

Did you know?
The *roots* of asparagus increase mental acuity and inhibit mental disorders. They are a diuretic and increase breast milk secretion. Juice or powder made from asparagus roots is used in the treatment of biliary colic, biliousness, haemoptysis, piles, diarrhoea, rheumatic fever, nervous debility, insomnia and high blood pressure, and can also be eaten to improve a generally run-down condition.

❊ Avocados

– have the highest vitamin E content of all fruits and are rich in proteins

TASTE sweet
ELEMENT earth

Nutritional value
- rich in phosphorus, sulphur and chlorine
- high vitamin E content in the fruit oil
- high content of iron and copper, potassium and sodium

Did you know?
Avocados contain everything a human body needs apart from vitamin C. (Only olives contain a comparable amount of fat.) The vitamin A they contain maintains a resistance against bacterial infection.

The exceptionally high amount of fat (25–30 per cent) will over-stimulate the gall bladder if you eat too many, because as soon as you eat fat, bile rushes into the duodenum.

Avocados are useful for people who want to increase weight: eat 1–2 a day. The sugars can be directly absorbed with minimal digestion.

The protein in an avocado is superior to cereal protein. The pulp of the fruit can be mixed with water and used as a substitute for milk. It is fibreless and makes a fine emulsion. It can safely be given to babies. In quality the avocado is superior to meat because it is free of bacteria. If you desire longevity, include avocados in your diet.

Beneficial in the treatment of
- digestive disorders
- auto-intoxication
- colitis, biliousness
- halitosis
- intestinal putrefaction – remember, it contains no bacteria
- hyperacidity and sour stomach – use well-ripened papaya with avocado as a basic diet
- duodenitis
- gall bladder diseases

- duodenal ulcers – because they are soothing to the membranes and pass quickly into the intestines

✳ Bananas (plantains)

– protect the mucus lining of the stomach; anti-ulcerous

TASTE sweet
ELEMENT earth

Nutritional value
- rich in potassium, calcium, magnesium, phosphorus, sulphur, iron and copper
- contain vitamins A, B, C, E, G

Did you know?
The banana is similar to the potato in that it has a high caloric value. Use green plantains for cooking. Bananas have an anti-ulcerous effect. Their healing effect is enhanced when they are overripe and have black spots, but the skin must be undamaged. Their starches are converted into sugars. The inside skin is the most potent part and combats bacteria. It is high in vitamin P (bioflavanoids).

Together with yoghurt, bananas are useful to restore the flora of the colon and to combat candida and the side effects of antibiotics. Bananas are food for the 'friendly' *acidophilus* bacteria in our intestines, particularly when combined with natural yoghurt.

The juice of the outer fibre is said to be an antidote against snakebites, including cobra venom, when administered immediately.

Tea made from plaintain leaves can be used to strengthen the eyes.

Natural therapeutic effect
- stomachic

Beneficial in the treatment of
- ulcers of stomach and duodenum – the banana diet is one of the most powerful diets for ulcers. Bananas neutralize the stomach acid and thicken the mucus lining of the stomach. They should be a regular part of the recovery process after an ulcer has been diagnosed to prevent re-occurring damage.

- diarrhoea
- dysentery
- typhoid fever
- anaemia
- acidosis
- diabetes – because of their high content of easy-to-absorb sugars
- high blood cholesterol (a banana contains as much pectin as an apple)

Caution

When you buy a banana ensure that the skin is not damaged. If it is, unwelcome bacteria can enter the fruit.

❁ Barley

– diuretic, anti-allergic; kidney tonic

TASTE sweet
ELEMENT earth

Nutritional value
- rich in potassium, silicon, iron and phosphoric acid

Did you know?

The partially germinated and dried grain of barley is a source of malt. Malt helps convert starch into dextrin and sugar, assisting the digestion of starchy and floury foods.

Natural therapeutic effects
- demulcent (soothes), diuretic

Beneficial in the treatment of
- weakness of the kidneys
- diseases of the urinary system, eg cystitis
- anaemia
- constipation
- high blood cholesterol due to beta glucan

Barley flour can be used to replace wheat products in breads, cakes and pasta. It is best to use wholemeal barley, freshly ground at home if possible. Cooked barley can be used as an external application for sores and tumours.

❈ Beans

– rich in proteins; rich in iron and zinc

TASTE astringent
ELEMENT water

Adzuki beans

There are 60 different kinds of beans, including black beans, black-eyed beans, chick peas, kidney beans, mung beans, split peas, white beans, brown beans and soya beans.

Nutritional value
- rich in potassium, calcium and phosphorus
- rich in iron (especially black beans)
- rich in proteins

Did you know?
Recent research has shown that beans may be a factor in preventing cancer and heart disease because they contain isoflovones, which act like a shield to prevent oestrogen from invading cells. Isoflovones play a role in protecting the body from oestrogen-dependent tumours in the breasts and ovaries.

Caution
To improve your digestion of proteins, add asafoetida (gum powder), cumin seeds (whole and ground) and fresh coriander to your bean dishes. Always add salt after the beans have cooked.

Natural therapeutic effect
- diuretic

Beneficial in the treatment of
- high cholesterol
- cancer
- dropsy
- sciatica

- chronic rheumatism
- kidney and urinary problems
- uric acid accumulation
- loss of <u>albumin</u> via the urine during pregnancy

see page 140 204

❊ Beetroot

– rebuilds red blood cells (highly recommended for anaemia); good for bulk (alleviates constipation)

TASTE sweet
ELEMENT earth

Nutritional value
- rich in potassium, sodium, calcium, magnesium, phosphorus, sulphur and silicon, some iron
- high in vitamin A

Did you know?
You can also eat the beet leaves. They are delicious steamed.

Natural therapeutic effect
- nerve tonic

Beneficial in the treatment of
- calcium deposits – it is an excellent solvent
- heart troubles caused by thickened arteries
- varicose veins
- diseases of kidneys and liver
- gallstones
- jaundice
- gout
- lumbago
- constipation
- <u>anaemia</u>
- suppressed menstruation
- low haemoglobin

❉ Black salt

– contains <u>sulphur</u> which acts on the liver; carminative

TASTE pungent
ELEMENT water

Nutritional value
• high content of sulphur

Did you know?
Black salt comes from India. It can usually be found in Asian and Indian stores. Sulphur is a strong blood cleanser. This salt is a useful additive to almost all fruit and vegetable juices in place of white salt. <u>When a salt-free diet is recommended, use black salt in moderation</u>, but you may need to overcome your resistance to its '<u>rotten egg</u>' smell.   ←

Natural therapeutic effects
• eliminative, blood-purifying

❉ Blackcurrants

– reduce the ageing of brain cells; a remedy for diarrhoea

TASTE sweet
ELEMENT earth

Did you know?
This berry contains anthocyanosides, which destroy the intestinal bacteria *E. coli* that cause diarrhoea. Anthocyanosides block the ability of cholesterol to stick to artery walls. Latest scientific speculation suggests that anthocyanosides interact with collagen in the blood vessels to create tough and elastic walls which can withstand the cholesterol.

Natural therapeutic effects
• astringent, tonic

Beneficial in the treatment of
• diarrhoea

- enteritis
- chronic appendicitis
- leucorrhoea
- high blood cholesterol

✳ Bran

– important for bulk, as well as for the minerals it provides

TASTE astringent
ELEMENT wood

Did you know?

Bran or husk is the name for the outer covering of grains. Since it contains large amounts of minerals, it should not be thrown away. The German healer, Kneipp, discovered that the husk is more valuable than the grain itself. Wheat bran contains more proteins, fat, minerals, fibre, calcium, magnesium, phosphorus, iron, potassium, copper, chlorine, vitamin A, thiamine, riboflavin, choline and panthenal than the wheat grain. Grain is more acidic without the bran. Wheat protein is inferior in quality to bran protein and lacks many of the essential amino acids which are found in the bran. Bran is the main source of iron for the human body. If we eat food from which the bran has been removed, our bodies suffer from a serious loss of iron, which is difficult to make up for in other foods. The consequences of this deficiency are constipation, digestive disturbances and nutritional disorders. (Wholewheat bread contains twice as much iron as white bread.)

Natural therapeutic effect

- nerve tonic

Beneficial in the treatment of

- anaemia – nervous and anaemic people benefit from bran tea. Bran baths can also be used to soothe irritations of the skin.
- diabetes – the bran of sesame seeds is very good for diabetics because it removes starch from the blood.

❇ Broccoli

– combats outbursts of herpes; high amount of zinc improves production of red blood cells; anti-colon cancer

TASTE sweet
ELEMENT earth

Nutritional value
- abundant in vitamin A and beta carotene, vitamin C, zinc, potassium
- high in chlorophyll

Did you know?
Broccoli belongs to the cruciferous family of plants which also includes cauliflowers, watercress and Brussels sprouts. All cruciferous plants are rich in iron and vitamin K.

Broccoli is very rich in zinc. Zinc and iron are interrelated and are both needed for the production of red blood cells. Anaemic people who take iron artificially find that it creates constipation. Broccoli by contrast produces more blood in the system. It also works as roughage.

Recent research has shown that broccoli contains a photochemical called sulfophane. This triggers the body's production of the enzymes that protect a cell's DNA from damage. Broccoli also contains dithiolthiones, which stimulate the body to fight cancer. That makes broccoli a number one cancer fighter when eaten daily. Broccoli is best eaten together with a protein – and *never overcook* it. This is the optimum combination to help convey amino acids to the brain.

Natural therapeutic effects
- anticatarrhal, anticancerous; strengthens the immune system

Beneficial in the treatment of
- anaemia – as a dietary supplement

❋ Cabbage

– *miracle cure for stomach ulcers (in combination with potatoes)*

TASTE sweet
ELEMENT earth

Nutritional value
- rich in sulphur (produces lots of wind!)
- vitamins U, C

Did you know?
It is important to cook cabbage in its own juice and to chop it <u>fine</u> to make it more digestible. Raw cabbage juice contains vitamin U which is destroyed in cooking. Cabbage juice from the stem is an excellent remedy for ulcers. The Romans and Egyptians knew the value of cabbage in preventing intoxication. They would drink the juice before a big diner and chew cabbage seeds to avoid hangovers and sickness from overconsumption of alcohol.

Raw cabbage juice is beneficial in the treatment of
- acidosis
- gout
- rheumatism
- ulcers
- infected ulcers
- boils and carbuncles
- spots and blisters
- psoriasis
- headaches and migraine
- neuralgia
- rheumatism
- burns
- cerebral inflammation
- asthma
- cystitis
- sprains
- bronchitis

The juice drained from sauerkraut is very effective for generating bowel movements and stimulating the body. It contains lactic acid, which acts as a disinfectant in the colon.

If you suffer from any of the following, eat 500g of cabbage daily.

- diabetes
- rheumatism
- asthma
- digestive disorders

Cabbage leaves, washed and warmed, can be used as a poultice or compress on the affected area. They will attract any toxic matter which has accumulated in the skin.

Caution

Red cabbage in large amounts is not healthy. The significant amounts of iron it contains create constipation and irritation. This is true for most red vegetables. Red beetroot is the exception.

FRESH JUICE RECIPE

For a stomach ulcer, mix:

- 25ml potato juice
- 25ml cabbage juice

Drink immediately, on an empty stomach.

❋ Calendula

– heals wounds and sprains

Natural therapeutic effects

- antispasmodic, aperient, cholagogic, diaphoretic, vulnerary

Beneficial in the treatment of

- gastro-intestinal problems
- fevers
- boils and abscesses
- vomiting
- wounds
- sprains
- pulled muscles
- sores

✻ Camomile

– *relaxes the stomach*

TASTE sweet
ELEMENT earth

Nutritional value
- contains iron, calcium, magnesium, potassium
- vitamin A

Natural therapeutic effects
- anodyne, antispasmodic, aromatic, bitter tonic, stimulant, stomachic

Camomile tea is beneficial in the treatment of
- flatulence
- dyspepsia
- fever
- restlessness in children

Use camomile oil externally to treat
- sores and wounds
- colic
- spasms
- stomach cramps
- swellings
- painful joints

✻ Camphor

– *opens the nasal passages and expels catarrh; also used in oils for the ligaments*

SMELL astringent
ELEMENT metal

Did you know?
Camphor is available as oil or crystals. Crushed camphor crystals are very helpful for breathing difficulties.

Natural therapeutic effect
- anticatarrhal

Beneficial in the treatment of
- colds and flu
- bronchitis

❈ Cardamoms

– help food digestion

TASTE astrigent
ELEMENT metal

Did you know?
Indians chew cardamons to sweeten and refresh the breath. They are also eaten as an aphrodisiac – black cardamons for men, green cardamoms for women.

Natural therapeutic effects
- appetizing, carminative, stimulant, stomachic

Beneficial in the treatment of
- digestive problems
- stomach acid

❈ Carrots

– contain large amounts of beta carotene; favourable for eye disorders and lung troubles; good for skin rashes; a multi-healer

TASTE sweet
ELEMENT earth

Nutritional value
- rich in vitamin A, contains vitamins B, C, and E
- contain large doses of calcium which is good for hair and nails
- rich in potassium, sulphur, sodium, phosphorus and iron

Did you know?

In oriental healing carrots are the food for the liver. The sense organ related to the liver is the eyes. Carrots are always best eaten raw because the minerals and vitamins they contain are destroyed in cooking. The high content of beta carotene makes carrots especially valuable for sufferers of diseases of the mucous membranes, the lungs and the skin. One carrot a day is a healthy supplement, especially for smokers.

Natural therapeutic effects
- anthelmintic, carminative, diuretic, stimulant

Beneficial in the treatment of
- failing eyesight
- deteriorating complexion
- unhealthy skin, hair and nails
- colds
- diarrhoea – also in infants
- derangements of liver and biliary digestion
- nervous conditions
- anaemia
- ulcerous conditions
- jaundice
- cancer, especially of the lungs and pancreas

Carrot seeds are used as an aphrodisiac and nerve tonic, and to induce abortion.

❋ Cassia (senna)

– inner part of the cinnamon plant, which has a warming effect on the body

TASTE pungent
ELEMENT fire

Did you know?

The cinnamon plant grows in India and Pakistan. Cassia is the inner part; the outer part is the cinnamon bark (see separate entry).

Natural therapeutic effects
- highly antiparasitic, tonic, purgative, expectorant, astringent

As an ointment made with Vaseline or lanoline, is beneficial in the treatment of
- herpes and other parasitic skin diseases
- insect bites
- eczema

As a tea, is useful to counteract
- halitosis and bad taste in the mouth – use as a mouth wash
- chronic constipation
- ringworm

Caution
Do not use for haemorrhoids or inflammation of the alimentary canal.

❀ Cauliflower

– combats cancer; clears liver congestion

TASTE sweet
ELEMENT earth

Nutritional value
- rich in sulphur

Did you know?
Cauliflower belongs to the family of cruciferous vegetables, and is therefore powerful in combating cancer (but because cauliflower lacks chlorophyll, broccoli is the preferred vegetable). Most of the minerals are in the green leaves. Use them in soups or steamed. They are very nutritious.

Natural therapeutic effect
- anticancerous

Beneficial in the treatment of
- cancer

- ulcers – when taken with potatoes in juice form
- arthritic pains – when applied as a poultice

❋ Cayenne

– activates the immune system to kill germs; blood purifier; very rich in vitamin C

TASTE hot
ELEMENT metal

Nutritional value
- rich in vitamins A, B, C and PABA
- builds up resistance

Did you know?
Chilli pepper raises the body temperature, thereby killing many toxins.

Chillies stimulate the body's production of endorphins – you can experience a natural 'high' after eating them. If you are not used to eating chillies, start by eating small amounts, and make sure you have some yoghurt to cool your taste buds. Your level of tolerance will grow as you keep eating them. Try tabasco if you really dislike eating fresh chillies.

Natural therapeutic effects
- appetizing, digestive, irritant, anti-ulcerous, stimulant, tonic, anti-cancerous

Beneficial in the treatment of
- high blood cholesterol
- stomach and bowel pains and cramps

In tincture form, is useful for
- toothache – it acts as a pain killer
- rheumatism
- arthritis
- pleuritis
- pericarditis

Caution

Excessive consumption can cause gastro-enteritis and kidney damage. Not advisable for children.

❋ Celery

– great blood cleanser; dissolves calcium deposits

TASTE sweet
ELEMENT earth

Nutritional value
- rich in zinc
- rich in vitamins A, G
- rich in sodium, potassium, sulphur

Did you know?
The high content of sodium keeps calcium and magnesium in liquid form, thus inhibiting crystal formation. Celery is therefore very useful for people suffering from arthritis since it disperses calcium deposits.

Because of its sobering effect it is useful for hangovers.

Celery is best used in fresh juice form. It is often recommended in the Health Manual (Part II of this book).

Natural therapeutic effects
- anti-inflammatory, anti-arthritic/rheumatic, blood-purifying, carminative, stomachic

Seeds

Nutritional value
- rich in iron and vitamins A, B, and C

Beneficial in the treatment of
- arthritis
- muscle spasms
- liver problems
- high blood pressure

Make a tea from the seeds (1 teaspoon per cup) or chew the seeds thoroughly and swallow them with a cup of hot water.

❋ Chives

– free the lungs and help to expel mucus

TASTE pungent
ELEMENT metal

Nutritional value
- rich in potassium, calcium, sulphur
- contain iron and arsenic

Did you know?
Chives belong to the allium family, as do leeks, spring onions and onions. They are best used in salads with spring onions and other greens.

Natural therapeutic effects
- appetizing, digestive, antioxidant

Beneficial in the treatment of
- catarrhal conditions
- anaemia

❋ Cider vinegar

– reduces acidity

TASTE sour
ELEMENT wood

Nutritional value
Cider vinegar is packed with essential amino acids and helpful vitamins, minerals, and enzymes. It is also very rich in magnesium.

Did you know?
Cider vinegar is a universal preservative and a general purpose remedy.

When vinegar is made from fresh natural apples it contains a healthy dose of pectin. As pectin works its way through the digestive system, cholesterol becomes bound to it and is then eliminated from the body. Less cholesterol in the body reduces the risk of cardiovascular problems, heart attacks and strokes.

Taken *internally*, by drinking 3 teaspoons with 1 tablespoon honey in a cup of hot water 1–3 times a day, cider vinegar can:

- fight germs generally
- balance alkalinity and acidity
- cut grease
- relieve pain of varicose veins
- disperse headaches
- kill infection
- soothe sore throats
- control the appetite (helpful for weight loss)
- minimize memory loss
- eliminate calcium deposits (useful for people suffering from gout and arthritis)

For skin troubles, to fade age spots and to treat eczema, put 1 cup of cider vinegar, together with Epsom salts or mustard bath salts, in your bath.

Caution
Cider or fermented apple juice can suppress the blood's ability to dissolve clots, which means that it may clot more easily. Fresh apple juice by contrast does not have this effect.

❋ Cinnamon (bark)

– *warming and diuretic*

TASTE astringent
ELEMENT metal

Did you know?
Cinnamon bark is an ingredient of the famous Tiger Balm, which gives relief from all sorts of pain – headache, toothache and rheumatic and

arthritic pains. Cinnamon is also used in barley water because of its warming and diuretic attributes.

Natural therapeutic effects
- diuretic, anti-inflammatory, anticatarrhal, astringent, carminative, stimulant

❋ Cloves

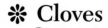

– anaesthetic, used with toothache

TASTE astringent
ELEMENT metal

Natural therapeutic effects
- anodyne, anti-emetic, antiseptic, anaesthetic

Beneficial in the treatment of
- nausea and vomiting
- flatulence
- digestion problems
- acid stomach
- toothache

Cloves are a favourite remedy for toothache. Chew 3–4 cloves or apply clove oil to numb the area and soothe the nerves of the tooth.

❋ Coconuts

– contain caprilic acid which is antibacterial and antifungal; the milk is similar to human milk

TASTE sweet
ELEMENT earth

Nutritional value
- contain vitamins A, B and some C
- very high in potassium, sodium, chlorine

Did you know?

The flesh of the coconut contains 70 per cent fat. Coconut milk has a chemical base similar to that of mother's milk. When taken fresh, it is a complete protein nutriment. It contains all the amino-acids and ranks highly as a digestive milk. Coconut milk is therefore particularly beneficial during pregnancy.

The milk of the green coconut is a rich source of mineral salts and vitamins, especially C and most B complexes.

Natural therapeutic effects
• blood-purifying, diuretic

Beneficial in the treatment of
• flatulence
• urinary diseases
• vomiting
• general weakness
• dyspepsia
• nervousness
• fatigue

❋ Comfrey

– used for fractures; treatment for worms

TASTE astringent
ELEMENT earth

Nutritional value
• rich in calcium
• contains phosphorus, potassium
• vitamins A, C and E

Did you know?

The use of comfrey has been linked to cancer, and its root is no longer available because of possible health dangers. The problem appears to be caused by the alkaloid *purrolizidehe*, which affects the liver tissue. Tea made from the plant is effective in helping to heal bone fractures.

Comfrey is preferably used as a homoeopathic remedy called symphytum.

Beneficial in the treatment of
- broken bones
- swellings
- cramps
- coughs and asthma

It is also useful where there is a calcium deficiency.

❋ Coriander

– used fresh, it adds a distinctive flavour to cooking; seeds fried in oil become sour and tasty

TASTE astrigent
ELEMENT metal

Coriander is a delicious herb when eaten fresh. It can also be eaten dried and the seeds can be used as a condiment.

Natural therapeutic effects
- antispasmodic, appetizing, aromatic, carminative, stomachic, diuretic

In dried form, coriander is beneficial in the treatment of
- flatulent colic
- rheumatism
- neuralgia
- conjunctivitis – use as an eye-wash
- ulcerations of the mouth and throat – use the seeds
- chronic ulcers and carbuncles – use in a poultice

✳ Cos (Romaine) lettuce

– reduces hypertension, aids gastric disorders, heart palpitations, nervousness; induces sound sleep

TASTE bitter
ELEMENT fire

Nutritional value
- rich in zinc, chlorophyll, iron, magnesium, calcium, phosphorus
- contains vitamins A, B and E
- contains natural opiates

Did you know?
Cos lettuce contains good quantities of minerals and vitamins, but not many calories, so is a good antidote to obesity. A portion of lettuce and lemon juice before a meal diminishes the appetite and reduces any craving for oily foods.

Cos (Romaine) lettuce was part of the 'basic natural remedy kit' of the Bohemians – the Romanies – together with garlic, onions, ginger, lemons, chillies and hot peppers.

Made into a soup, cos lettuce is ideal for hypertension. It has a soothing effect on the nervous system because of opiate-like substances present in the outer leaves. It also aids against gastric and digestive upsets and intestinal problems.

Beneficial in the treatment of
- diabetes
- anaemia
- acidity
- hypertension
- insomnia
- headaches
- urinary disorders
- nervousness and heart palpitations

❈ Cranberries

– fresh juice is useful for bladder infections and kidney problems

TASTE sour
ELEMENT wood

Nutritional value
- rich in calcium, sulphur and chlorine
- high in vitamin A

Did you know?
Because cranberries contain large amounts of oxalic acid, they should not be eaten raw.

Both whole cranberries and their juice increase the acid in urine which kills the bacteria that cause infection. They appear to create a coating around hostile bacteria and germs, making it difficult for them to stick to the body's internal surfaces.

Natural therapeutic effects
- germ-killing, antibacterial

Beneficial in the treatment of
- diarrhoea
- infections of the urinary tract – bladder, kidney, prostate, urethra

❈ Cucumber

– removes uric acid from blood; diuretic; cooling in summer

TASTE sweet
ELEMENT earth

Nutritional value
- high in potassium, phosphorus, iron, silicon and calcium

Did you know?
Combined with carrots, beets and celery, cucumber juice is especially beneficial for rheumatic conditions. It dissolves uric acid accumulations

which form kidney stones and gall bladder stones. Cucumbers give immediate relief when there is a burning sensation in the stomach.

If you suffer from hyperacidity, a gastric ulcer or duodenal ulcer, cucumber juice works wonders. Drink 100–150ml every 2 hours.

Natural therapeutic effects
- diuretic, laxative, aperient

Useful as a
- digestive aid
- bowel cleanser

❉ Cumin

– aids digestion

TASTE astringent
ELEMENT metal

Did you know?
Cumin powder is carminative (relieves flatulence). It is needed to balance any fresh juices containing beetroot, which can otherwise be too earthy to digest.

There are three varieties of cumin – black, white, and Kashmiri black – each of which has different properties.

Black cumin or black jeera is very aromatic, diuretic, anthelmintic, carminative and stimulant. A powder of the seeds mixed with sesame oil can be applied locally on eruptive diseases.

Natural therapeutic effects
- stomachic, diuretic, carminative, stimulant, astringent, emmenagogic

Beneficial in the treatment of
- flatulence
- dyspepsia
- diarrhoea

❋ Dandelion

– strengthens the liver; tea good for digestion

TASTE bitter
ELEMENT fire

Nutritional value
- the leaves are high in vitamin A (at least 7 times more than carrots), vitamins B1, C and G
- rich in sodium, calcium and potash, chlorophyll

Did you know?
Dandelion leaves are most tasty in spring, when the leaves are young and soft. The root can be eaten raw after being grated. It contains pectin, sugar and levulin. Roasted dandelion roots are a refreshing alternative to coffee, and a lot healthier!

Natural therapeutic effects
- aperient, cholagogic, diuretic, stomachic, tonic

Beneficial in the treatment of
- obstructions of the stomach, liver, gall and spleen
- liver problems – acts as a hepatic stimulant
- dyspepsia
- jaundice
- dropsy
- chronic skin diseases
- hypochondria
- gout and rheumatism

Dandelion can be used as a blood tonic and to remove poisons from the body. It is also effective for removing excess water from the body in oedematous conditions which have been caused by liver problems

❊ Echinacea

– strengthens the immune system; good for skin problems

TASTE bitter
ELEMENT fire

Did you know?
North America Indians used this herb for wounds, snakebites and abscesses.

Natural therapeutic effects
• antiseptic, depurative, digestive, blood-purifying

Beneficial in the treatment of
• influenza
• eczema
• acne
• boils that indicate contaminants in the blood

Caution
Do not use during pregnancy or for multiple sclerosis, tuberculosis, or collagen disorders.

❊ Endive

– purifies the blood and stimulates appetite

TASTE bitter
ELEMENT fire

Nutritional value
• contains potassium, magnesium, chlorine, sodium, calcium, phosphorus, sulphur and iron
• contains vitamins A, C and G

Did you know?
Endive is related to the dandelion family. It is a good substitute for cos (Romaine) lettuce. The endive has very little nutritional value other than

its bitterness. All foods which are bitter are blood purifiers. Bitter foods also stimulate the production of saliva. It is used as an appetiser, especially in France, where it is eaten to balance the effects of wine. Endive is beneficial as a general body cleanser.

Natural therapeutic effects
• mineralizing, blood-purifying

❈ Eucalyptus

– oil is inhaled to open congested nasal passages; used as a gargle to clear the throat

TASTE astringent
ELEMENT metal

Natural therapeutic effects
• antiseptic, deodorant, expectorant, stimulant

Beneficial in the treatment of
• lung diseases
• colds
• sore throats
• asthma
• bronchitis
• pyorrhoea
• burns

❈ Euphrasia

– for all eye troubles

TASTE bitter
ELEMENT fire

Did you know?
For centuries the healing effect of euphrasia on the eyes has been common knowledge. For this reason it is also called eyebright.

Natural therapeutic effects
- astringent, tonic

Beneficial in the treatment of
- eye inflammations
- eyestrain and other eye problems

❋ Evening primrose

– for pain relief and hormonal balance

TASTE sweet
ELEMENT earth

Nutritional value
- contains linolenic acid, vitamin F, and more GLA (gamma linolenic acid) than any other food source

Did you know?
The body does not produce GLA; it must be provided in food.

Natural therapeutic effects
- astringent, mucilaginous

Beneficial in the treatment of
- mental depression
- coughs and colds
- PMS (pre-menstrual syndrome)
- general weakness
- rheumatic conditions
- inflammation

Evening primrose is also effective for pain relief, blood purification, and as a stimulant for the liver, spleen and digestive system.

❊ Fennel

– for relaxation and relief for digestive system

TASTE sweet
ELEMENT earth

Did you know?

Fennel is an essential herb for mothers with new-born babies: it stimulates the milk flow in those who are breastfeeding, and 1 teaspoonful of fennel tea relieves the baby's stomach-ache.

Natural therapeutic effects

- leaves – diuretic, digestive, appetizing, lactagogic, stimulant, aromatic
- seeds – sweetening, laxative, aphrodisiac, stomachic, anthelmintic, carminative, diuretic

Beneficial in the treatment of

- eye diseases
- burning sensations
- fever
- thirst
- wounds
- dysentery
- biliousness
- diseases of the chest, spleen and kidneys
- headaches
- amenorrhoea
- stomach-ache in children
- flatulence

Fennel is also beneficial after chemotherapy and radiation treatments.

✻ Fenugreek

*– clears entire digestive tract after poisoning; used for
diarrhoea; good for diabetics*

TASTE bitter
ELEMENT fire

Did you know?

The seeds contain several alkaloids, which stimulate the appetite via the
nervous system. These alkaloids are rich in phosphates, lecithin and neu-
cleo-albumin. Fenugreek can be used as a substitute for codliver oil in the
treatment of lymphatism, scrofula, rickets, anaemia, neurasthenia, gout
and diabetes. The recommended dose is 2 teaspoons of powdered seeds
taken daily in broth, milk or jam.

You can also soak 2 teaspoons of seeds overnight and eat them with
salads or soup or any meal. This is a good way to prevent diabetes, especially if you know you are prone to the illness because of hereditary or
lifestyle factors.

Natural therapeutic effects

- aromatic, aphrodisiac, astringent, carminative, demulcent, diuretic,
  emmenagogic, emollient, lactagogic, nutritive, tonic

Beneficial in the treatment of

- dyspepsia with loss of appetite
- diarrhoea
- dysentery
- colic
- flatulence
- rheumatism
- enlargement of the liver and spleen
- chronic coughs
- dropsy
- vomiting from slight food poisoning

REMEDIES

Ground seeds are said to be able to minimize hair loss and promote the
growth of hair when applied to the head as a paste.

In cases of leucorrhoea, pessaries made of fenugreek powder are beneficial for the uterus and vagina.

For sore throats, gargle with 1 teaspoon fenugreek powder in a cup of water.

Poultices made with fenugreek powder can be used to dissolve swellings painlessly in the treatment of gout, neuralgia, sciatica, swollen glands, wounds, carbuncles, fistulas and skin irritations. They can also be used to treat wounds on the feet.

In tea form, useful to counteract
- indigestion
- bilious disorders
- flatulence
- a sluggish liver

❋ Feverfew

– the remedy for migraine

TASTE bitter
ELEMENT fire

Did you know?
2–3 fresh leaves chewed with a piece of bread will help overcome headaches.

Natural therapeutic effects
- carminative, emmenagogic, purgative, stimulant, tonic

In powdered form, benificial in the treatment of
- migraine
- colic
- flatulence
- indigestion
- colds

It is also used to increase the fluidity of mucus in the lungs and bronchial tubes.

❋ Figs

– highly alkaline; reduce tumours; a good laxative

TASTE sweet
ELEMENT earth

Natural therapeutic effects
- demulcent, emollient, laxative

Did you know?
Fresh roasted figs are a good healing agent in a poultice for boils, tumours and haemorrhoids. Figs can also be used to soothe the mucous membranes of the respiratory system. The milky juice that comes out of the stem of the fresh fruit is used to treat warts.

Because figs have an effect on the liver and gall bladder, (which are connected to the eyes in the Chinese meridian system), they are also used to improve the eyesight.

The most potent part of the fig is the juice. The effective agent in the fig is benzaldehyde, which is anticancerous. It also contains ficin, an enzyme that aids digestion.

It is reported that figs can absorb pollution in the air.

Beneficial in the treatment of
- constipation
- cancer
- gangrene
- haemorrhoids

Figs are also used to:
- reduce body heat
- lubricate the intestines
- kill bacteria
- heal inflammation and swelling
- build muscles

❋ Garlic

– a general tonic; clears catarrh and coughs

TASTE pungent
ELEMENT metal

Nutritional value
- contains vitamins B and C, some vitamin A
- rich in calcium, sulphur, zinc, copper, potassium and phosphoric acid

Did you know?
Garlic is a natural antibiotic. It has strong germ-killing powers. Garlic stimulates the activity of all the digestive organs. Because of its anti-catarrhal qualities, garlic is good for respiratory problems. Garlic regularizes the functioning of the liver and gall bladder. It is helpful for all intestinal infections and for problems caused by putrefactive intestinal bacteria. Garlic lowers the blood pressure and stimulates circulation and the action of the heart.

Poultices applied over the abdomen heal gastric intestinal catarrh. For sexual debility and impotence, especially for older men, garlic treatment is very effective.

Garlic can be applied externally on warts. It can be used as a healing agent for numerous diseases, and will prevent constipation if eaten regularly. As a killer of various bacteria, garlic works best when eaten raw. Views on the number of cloves required to prevent illness range from half a clove to 18 cloves a day, eaten raw.

Note: The smell of garlic on the breath can be counteracted by chewing parsley, cardamom seeds or an apple, or by washing the mouth out with lemon juice.

Natural therapeutic effects
- stimulant, diaphoretic, expectorant, diuretic, aphrodisiac, tonic
- antifungal, anticatarrhal, antibacterial, antiprotozoan, antiparasitic, antioxidant, antithrombotic,
- lowers blood cholesterol, strengthens the immune system

Beneficial in the treatment of
- problems of the digestive system such as excessive stomach acidity

- pneumonia and tuberculosis
- acute and chronic bronchitis
- chronic stomach and intestinal catarrh
- dysentery
- cholera
- typhoid and parathyroid fever
- worms

❊ Ginger

– essential for healing; good for increasing the local blood flow

TASTE pungent
ELEMENT metal

Did you know?
Fresh ginger is a superb healer, and has been long used as such in the East. It can be used as a paste made from dried ginger, or in powder form. For headaches, it can disperse the pain in less than 15 minutes.

Ginger contains gingerol, which has a similar effect to that of aspirin, and has the same blood-thinning qualities.

Natural therapeutic effects
- appetizing, carminative, diaphoretic, stimulant, antioxidant, diaphoretic, sialagogic, stimulant, antinauseous, anticoagulant

Beneficial in the treatment of
- dyspepsia
- colic
- vomiting
- diarrhoea – rub fresh ginger juice on and around the navel
- motion sickness – place a slice of ginger on your navel or suck a thick slice without chewing

RECIPE
For spasms of the stomach and intestines
Place 1 teaspoon grated ginger in a cup of boiling water. Add 20 drops soy sauce and a pinch of freshly ground black pepper. Leave for 10 minutes then drain and drink.

❋ Gourds

– contain an insulin-like substance; used as plant insulin in diabetes; good for purifying the blood; antimalarial

TASTE sweet
ELEMENT earth

Did you know?
Gourds are a type of cucumber. The bitter gourd (karela) is known to contain a 'plant insulin' which lowers the level of sugar in the blood and the urine. Diabetics should drink the juice of about 4 or 5 karelas every day between meals. You can easily grow them in your garden.

Natural therapeutic effects
• antibilious (bitter fruit), anthelmintic, laxative, tonic, stomachic

Beneficial in the treatment of
• jaundice
• rheumatism
• gout
• blood diseases
• anaemia
• urinary discharges
• asthma
• ulcers
• bronchitis
• diseases of the liver and spleen

❋ Grapefruit

– pink: rich in vitamins A and E; seeds are good for eliminating worms (vermifuge)

TASTE bitter sweet
ELEMENT water

Nutritional value
• rich in iron, vitamins B, C and, E – and A in smaller amounts

Did you know?

Grapefruit juice is most beneficial if you are feverish. It also helps against liver diseases and constipation. The fruit itself is a preventative against dysentery, diarrhoea, enteritis, typhus and infectious diseases of the digestive tract. The membranes and the pith contain pectin, which lowers cholesterol. Pink grapefruits are better than yellow ones because they contain more vitamin A.

If you have a tendency to diabetes, eat 3 grapefruits a day. Also, decrease your intake of starches, sweets and fats but eat more fruit and vegetables and drink more fresh juices.

❄ Grapes

– their highly nutritious value makes them an excellent fruit for
  monofasts to purify the entire body system

TASTE sweet
ELEMENT earth

Nutritional value
- large amount of potassium, low amount of sodium
- contain vitamins A, B1, B2, C and a large amount of glycids
- rich in pure glucose

Did you know?

Grapes are immensely valuable as a healing fruit (I recommended a grape diet in Chapter 1). They are rich in glucose, which is pure energy to the body. The glucose also supplies the heart with energy and strengthens the heart and its muscles. Grapes contain tartaric acid and malic acid. Tartaric acid stimulates the intestines.

As with many fruits, most of the benefits – minerals and vitamin B – are just under the skin. Grapes should be eaten, not just consumed as juice. The white grapes are richer in vitamins and are a better food in the morning. Red and black grapes are ideal as an evening meal. The high content of iron, copper and manganese makes the grape an excellent producer of haemoglobin. 250ml of grape juice once a day will help prevent secondary anaemia.

Because of the high content of potassium and water, the grape is a diuretic and thus good for kidney disorders. Grapes also stimulate hepatic and glycogenic functions and bile secretion. They also contain an element, similar to insulin, which is helpful in some kinds of diabetes.

Grapes also have a decalcifying effect.

Natural therapeutic effects
• demulcent, laxative, cooling, diuretic

Beneficial in the treatment of
• kidney troubles
• chronic and acute nephritis
• anaemia
• gout, rheumatism and arthritis – dissolve uric acid

RECIPE
For kidney and gall bladder stones, liver and urinary disorders
Boil 25g of vine leaves in 250ml of water and reduce to 125ml. Strain and add 25g of misri (Indian sugar candy). Drink every day.

❈ Green tea

– anticancerous; normalizes blood pressure; reduces damage from
nuclear radiation; beneficial in pregnancy

TASTE bitter
ELEMENT fire

Nutritional value
• rich in potassium and zinc
• rich in vitamins C, B1, B6, E and P

Did you know?
Green tea does not ferment and is therefore better than black tea because there are no by-products of fermentation (methylalcohol and ammonia, which can be damaging to the liver and eyesight).

In Japan, the land of green tea, many empirical studies have been conducted to attempt to prove the healing powers of green tea. Dr Hayashi became famous with his studies of green tea in connection with nuclear radiation. He discovered that green tea could partially block the absorption of strontium 90 and help the body to expel it via the alimentary system.

Natural therapeutic effects
- diuretic, anticancerous, stomachic, cardiac, antioxidant

Beneficial in the treatment of
- radiation
- cancer
- arteriosclerosis
- high blood pressure

Used to prevent:
- tooth decay
- strokes
- stomach problems and cancer

Because of the high amount of zinc it contains, green tea is particularly beneficial during pregnancy.

❋ Greens

– high in chlorophyll, which is essential for the production of red blood cells

TASTE bitter
ELEMENT water

Included here are green cabbage, the green part of leeks, the green leaves of kohlrabi, all green vegetables, and the green leaves of vegetables like beetroot, radishes, carrots and turnips.

Did you know?
All greens contain plenty of chlorophyll and minerals. Chlorophyll is the blood of plants. The difference between chlorophyll and haemoglobin is one oxygen molecule. When chlorophyll enters the body, it is converted into haemoglobin.

Natural therapeutic effect
- blood-building

Beneficial in the treatment of
- anaemia
- hypertension

❋ Hamamelis (witch hazel)

– mostly used as an ointment for wounds; used as tea for clearing eye fatigue; stops any kind of haemorrhage in the system, especially renal haemorrhage

Natural therapeutic effects
- astringent, homoeostatic, sedative, tonic

The leaves and bark are beneficial in the treatment of
- diarrhoea
- vaginitis
- haemorrhoids
- haemorrhages – especially renal
- insect bites
- bruises

Also used as
- a mouth and throat wash
- a poultice for eye inflammation
- an ointment for skin irritations

❋ Hawthorn

– heals weakened heart muscles

TASTE bitter
ELEMENT wood

Did you know?
Hawthorn regulates heart action and blood pressure, and increases the circulation of the heart muscle when it has been weakened by age or disease. It is therefore particularly helpful in combating heart failure in older people.

Natural therapeutic effects
• antispasmodic, cardiac, sedative, vasodilatory

Beneficial in the treatment of
• myocarditis
• arteriosclerosis
• nervous heart problems
• a weak heart

❋ Honey

– has outstanding antiseptic properties; heals second- and third-degree burns without leaving any scar tissue

TASTE sweet
ELEMENT earth

Nutritional value
• Honey consists of two kinds of sugar – dextrose and levulose. Dark honeys contain more minerals such as iron, copper and manganese than do light honeys.

Did you know?
Dextrose is very easily absorbed, whereas levulose is absorbed slowly – sometimes it is absorbed through the large intestines.

  Honey has the capacity to withdraw moisture from bacteria, causing them to die. But note that you can find these strong antiseptic qualities only in cold-pressed honey that does not contain additives. Heated honey loses its healing effect and can worsen a condition.

Natural therapeutic effects
• antiseptic, tonic

Beneficial in the treatment of
- athlete's foot – applied directly in between the toes, it can cure in 7–10 days
- ulcerated surfaces with pus
- cuts
- severe burns
- throat infections with difficulty in swallowing
- eye-troubles such as conjunctivitis, red eyes – dilute 1 teaspoon in a cup of water and insert 2 drops into the eyes with a dropper

Honey is also used as a laxative and a cough remedy, and to heal scars and restore strength after illness, especially heart disease.

✳ Horseradish (fresh)

– opens the lungs and frees nasal passages

TASTE pungent
ELEMENT metal

Did you know?
When used externally as a poultice or in a bath, horseradish stimulates blood flow.

Natural therapeutic effects
- diuretic, rubefacient, stomachic

Beneficial in the treatment of
- bladder infections
- gout and rheumatic problems
- lung problems
- coughs
- asthma
- colitis and intestinal problems

Caution
Consuming too much horseradish can produce diarrhoea or night-sweats.

❋ Juniper berries

– diuretic; useful for bladder infections

TASTE hot
ELEMENT fire

Did you know?
The diuretic quality of juniper berries is useful for reducing excess body water. They work particularly well when combined with barley. They are also useful where there is underproduction of hydrochloric acid.

Burning the berries and stems removes all kinds of bad smells from a room.

Natural therapeutic effects
• antiseptic, carminative, diuretic, rubefacient, stomachic, tonic

Beneficial in the treatment of
• gastro-intestinal infections, inflammations and cramps

Caution
Juniper berries can irritate the kidneys. Do not use them in large amounts if you suffer from kidney weakness.

❋ Lavender

– a multiple healer; can be inhaled; for headaches, fainting and dizziness

TASTE sweet
ELEMENT water

Natural therapeutic effects
• antispasmodic, carminative, cholagogic, diuretic, sedative, stimulant, stomachic, tonic

The essential oil is beneficial in the treatment of
• flatulence
• migraine headaches

- fainting
- dizziness
- putrefactive bacteria in the intestines

❋ Leeks

– clear the lungs of mucus; blood builder

TASTE pungent
ELEMENT metal

Did you know?
Leeks belong to the same allium family as garlic and onions and thus share most of their properties.

Leek and potato soup is very nourishing after a feverish illness.

Natural therapeutic effects
- antirheumatic, antiprostatic, skin-cleansing

❋ Lemons and Limes

– antiseptic and anti-inflammatory

TASTE sour
ELEMENT wood

Nutritional value
- rich in vitamins B and C

Natural therapeutic effects
- anticatarrhal, antiseptic, anti-acid, antifungal, antirash

Did you know?
Lemons and limes are used as a cure for influenza and colds, but they are also a remedy for acidosis (their alkaline content is 5 times greater than their acidic content), heartburn, rheumatism, dysentery, gout, sciatica, lumbago, neuralgia – all diseases which cause blood to be more acidic.

Because of its high potassium content, lemon juice is useful in dealing with heart weaknesses. Lemons are a powerful antiseptic, and are helpful for inflammation of the gums and to tighten loose teeth and render them white and shiny. Lemons destroy germs without destroying body tissue. Mixed with honey, their juice is a remedy for throat troubles. They can also stimulate corns to disappear when rubbed into them. The smell of lemons will keep mosquitoes out of your neighbourhood. Lemon rubbed into an aching back can relieve the pain.

Pure lemon juice also cleans the liver and, via the liver, improves eyesight and helps to restore muscular powers.

Beneficial in the treatment of
- gastric troubles
- worms
- piles
- boils
- asthma
- diabetes
- catarrh
- anaemia

Tips for overeaters and bulimics
Eat a slice of lemon before eating anything else.

❊ Lentils

– high in proteins, rich in iron

TASTE astringent
ELEMENT water

Nutritional value
- very high in protein (more than beans and peas)
- rich in iron and calcium

Did you know?
Lentils produce very little wind because they contain no sulphur. But they do contain uric acid and need to be properly cooked – without salt. You can use a few leaves of kombu to quicken the breakdown of proteins. Salt

should be added after the lentils are cooked. To improve digestion add some asafoetida, ginger and garlic to avoid fermentation.

All black lentils are rich in iron.

❄ Lily of the valley

– strengthens the heart

TASTE sweet
ELEMENT earth

Did you know?
This plant is used as a food in many Asian countries, particularly in China.

Natural therapeutic effects
• antispasmodic, cardiac, diuretic, laxative

Beneficial in the treatment of
• neurasthenia
• apoplexy
• epilepsy
• dropsy

Caution
In homoeopathy, lily of the valley is used as a cardiac drug. But if used excessively it tends to produce irregular heartbeats and stomach upsets.

❄ Linseed

– well-known for its laxative properties

TASTE sweet
ELEMENT earth

Natural therapeutic effects
• diuretic, emollient, laxative

Beneficial in the treatment of
- gonorrhoea
- gastro-intestinal disorders
- irritation of the genito-urinary organs
- nephritis
- cystitis
- colds and coughs
- sore chests and throats
- pulmonary complaints – use as a tea

REMEDY
Use the oil extract from the seeds as a laxative – 30–60ml a day.

❋ Kiwi fruit

– beneficial in early stages of diabetes, when eaten with the skin

TASTE sour
ELEMENT wood

Did you know?
Kiwis are the only known anti-diabetic fruit. When on a kiwi fast, eat at least 3kg a day. A 14-day fast will bring the sugar content of the blood and urine back to normal. To ensure that kiwi fruit do not produce blisters, they need to be ripe. Organic kiwis are best because it is important to eat the skin, which is rich in all minerals. To get rid of the not so tasty hairs, scrub the kiwis with a vegetable brush.

Beneficial in the treatment of
- diabetes
- weight problems

❋ Mackerel

– for cardiac troubles; has anti-ageing powers; rich in zinc

TASTE salty
ELEMENT water

Nutritional value
• rich in zinc
• rich in vitamin A

Did you know?
Mackerel and herring are a 'must' to combat ageing. Once you reach the age of 45, you should start eating mackerel. It contains omega 3 fish oils that are very powerful for healing, especially for cardiac difficulties.

Natural therapeutic effects
• antirheumatic, anti-arthritic, anticancerous, anti-inflammatory, antithrombotic

Beneficial in the treatment of
• migraine
• high blood pressure
• asthma
• psoriasis
• arteriosclerosis

Mackerel can also lower cholesterol levels and help to prevent heart attacks.

❋ Mangoes

– a complete fruit which contains everything; anti-infectious and delicious

TASTE sweet
ELEMENT earth

Nutritional values
- contain 6 times as much vitamin C as apples – the Langda mango, which is the richest in vitamin C, contains 83mg per 100g
- rich in vitamin A
- the peel contains at least the same amount of vitamins as the pulp; it is used for mango pickles in India

Did you know?
It is important that the mango is ripe. It provides the heart with tone, improves complexion, stimulates hunger and is helpful in liver disorders, loss of weight, dyspepsia and constipation. The kernel, bark and leaves (fresh and dried) are also used as remedies.

Mangoes are invigorating and fattening. Drinking mango juice is a rapid way to gain weight.

Beneficial in the treatment of
- defective vision
- sexual weaknesses
- neurasthenia
- kidney diseases

❋ Mint

– used to reduce tension in the digestive tract and for fevers and night-sweats

TASTE astringent
ELEMENT metal

Did you know?
There are many varieties of mint, including spearmint and applemint. Each has different properties. Mint has an effect on the liver and on digestion. It has a softening effect on hardened arteries, dissolves gravel in kidneys and the bladder, and can heal urticaria. For bad headaches place some mint on your forehead. It also reduces night-sweats. You can chop and sprinkle fresh mint on food, drink it as tea, or use the essential oil.

Natural therapeutic effects
- aromatic, carminative, stimulant, antispasmodic and stomachic, refrigerant

Beneficial in the treatment of
- insomnia
- cramps
- coughs
- migraine
- poor digestion
- nervous vomiting
- fevers – drink a cup of fresh mint tea

✳ Mushrooms

– lower LDL (low density lipoprotein) cholesterol and strengthen the immune system; tree ear mushrooms are good as a tonic

TASTE sweet
ELEMENT earth

Nutritional value
- rich in magnesium

Did you know?
Although most mushrooms contain little but water, provided you only wash them and do not remove the skin, they have certain healing powers. They are most effective when picked fresh from the woods – but it is important that you learn to identify them properly. Some mushrooms are very poisonous.

Shop-purchased button mushrooms are grown commercially and have no food value whatsoever.

In China some 200 types of mushrooms have been identified. The best known of these in the West are shiitake, oyster and tree ear (black fungus). They stimulate the immune system (antiviral), lower the blood cholesterol and are anticoagulant. They are therefore excellent in preventing heart attacks and strokes. Onion soup with Chinese mushrooms is useful in lowering blood pressure.

Natural therapeutic effects
- anticoagulant, cardiac, antiviral, antifungal, antibacterial

Beneficial in the treatment of
- high blood pressure

❋ Mustard

– blood purifier; assists in the production of red blood cells; used in a poultrice to reduce muscle pain

TASTE pungent
ELEMENT metal

Nutritional value
- richest source of food calcium
- rich in iron
- greens are rich in vitamin A, chlorophyll and zinc

Did you know?
We tend to use only the seeds, of which there are two kinds – yellow and black – but the leaves are also highly nutritious and delicious if prepared like spinach.

The *powder* can be used externally as a poultice. It helps to stimulate blood flow, and promotes healing in rheumatism, sciatica, peritonitis and neuralgia. 1 tablespoon of mustard powder added to the bath, with a little bicarbonate of soda and oil, will be revitalizing when fasting or when you have a cold or flu.

Natural therapeutic effects of seeds
- emetic, antiseptic, irritant, digestive

Beneficial in the treatment of
- intestinal stasis
- liver and stomach troubles
- weak heart muscles
- hair loss

Caution
Pure mustard oil irritates the skin, but mixed with alcohol (1 part oil, 4 parts alcohol) it can be used to activate blood flow.

REMEDY
Put 20–30 seeds in water and bring to the boil. Drink rapidly while it is still hot. The concoction will provoke vomiting, necessary after poisoning from toxins, alcohol and narcotics.

❋ Nettles

– blood cleanser with antiviral powers; good for arthritis

TASTE astringent
ELEMENT metal

Did you know?
The young spring leaves can be eaten raw. They are delicious in salads. After springtime the leaves must be cooked before being eaten. They may otherwise produce kidney damage.

Natural therapeutic effects
• astringent, diuretic, galactagogic, homoeostatic, tonic, antiviral

Beneficial in the treatment of
• blood in the urine
• haemorrhoids
• excessive menstrual flow
• urinary and rheumatic problems
• diarrhoea
• hair loss

Prevention

When you feel a cold or flu coming on, make this tasty soup with 500g red onions and plenty of fresh stinging nettles. Sauté them in a little oil with some fresh chillies, or lots of freshly ground pepper, then add 1½ litres of boiling water and let it reduce down to 1 litre. Add tamari (a type of soy sauce), nutmeg, cumin and some fresh coriander.

✻ Nutmeg

— valuable for withdrawal symptoms of drugs and hallucinogens; relaxes brain and nerves; good for inducing sleep

TASTE pungent and hot
ELEMENT metal

Did you know?

Nutmeg relaxes the brain and soothes the nerves when used in small quantities. In high doses it can produce double vision, stomach pains, delirium and other symptoms of poisoning.

Nutmeg helps to reduce withdrawal symptoms from cocaine and hallucinogens. It is commonly used in prisons when addicts have no access to drugs.

Natural therapeutic effects

- aromatic, carminative, hallucinogenic, stimulant

Beneficial in the treatment of

- colic
- flatulence
- fever
- exhaustion
- earache
- common colds
- cystitis
- insomnia
- gastric flu
- indigestion
- nausea
- travel sickness
- vomiting

RECIPE

For a relaxing drink, add the following to a glass of hot milk:

- 1 teaspoon cold-pressed honey
- ¼ teaspoon freshly ground nutmeg

❋ Nuts

– all nuts (except cashews) are rich in protein and fats

TASTE sweet and astringent
ELEMENT earth

Nutritional value
- contain mostly fat and protein
- rich in minerals
- source of vitamins B and E
- contain calcium phosphorus and potassium

Did you know?
Nuts must be chewed thoroughly to obtain the best effect. *Stale nuts are very dangerous* – they can produce food poisoning.

The protein content of nuts is equivalent to the protein content of fish. Most nuts contain unsaturated fats, *except* the coconut and the cashew nut which contain saturated fats.

Many people are allergic to *cashews*. The cashew nut contains 80 per cent starch – which is the reason for its sweet taste. The cashew nut is a starchy acid-producing fruit. Because it is rich in thiamine and other vitamin B complexes, it is useful for nervous weakness, indigestion, dyspepsia and loss of appetite. Regularly eaten it prolongs youth. Its high iron content suggests that it is useful in cases of anaemia. Cashews digest well with dried fruit. To experience their laxative quality eat 20 cashew nuts daily with a handful of raisins. The oil of cashew nuts is a useful anaesthetic, especially for psoriasis, warts, corns, ulcers and cracks in the feet.

Peanuts, cashews, pecans and *walnuts* are acid-forming – especially commercial peanut butter made from strongly roasted, heavily salted nuts. The peanut is now the least valuable of all nuts because it often carries fungus as a result of being grown in unnatural conditions for mass consumption. However, it has a quite astonishing healing effect on haemorrhages. A handful of roasted peanuts will provide good results in cases of excessive nose bleeding and heavy menstrual blood flow. Peanuts are difficult to digest unless they are chewed to a paste.

Almonds, hazelnuts and *Brazil* nuts are alkaline-forming. The *sweet chestnut* is also alkaline, but contains a much greater amount of starch and a small amount of protein and fat.

❋ Oils

— only cold-pressed oil has healing properties: it lowers LDL (low density lipoprotein) cholesterol and high blood pressure, and moves the bowels; the best oils are safflower, sunflower, sesame, canola and olive

TASTE sweet
ELEMENT earth

Did you know?

All *cold-pressed oils* are polyunsaturated, which is the healthiest form of oil. They help to lower the blood cholesterol and reduce the saturated fats in the blood which cause high blood pressure. Cold-pressed oil is very flavoursome.

The second best form of oil is heat-pressed. All other oils are mono-unsaturated or polyunsaturated.

Remember: if heated, use edible oils only once – reheated oils become saturated.

Apricot kernel and peach kernel oil

Peach and apricot kernel oil are anticancerous. They can be used as a sun shield to prevent skin cancer. While they are effective as a skin cancer preventative, they are of no benefit once skin cancer has been contracted. Hunza apricots are very rich in vitamin B17 and their kernels make an excellent breakfast.

Castor oil is a strong laxative but no good for cooking. It is liver-cleansing when used as a poultice. Lindelahr and Kneipp, both well-known water therapists, used castor oil for a hot-oil pack around the liver area, alternating with a cold body pack. The cold-drawn oil from the seeds of castor beans is medicinally the most useful part of the plant. It is an effective purgative when taken orally in cases of acute diarrhoea, especially if caused by food poisoning, or for constipation during pregnancy.

Coconut oil is rich in vitamins A and D and is used for skin diseases. It is also rich in caprilic acid, which can be an irritant, but is helpful against colonic infections.

Cod liver oil is rich in vitamins A and D.

Grapeseed oil is rich in arsenic – as are the pips of apples and pears and the seeds of watermelons and pumpkins. It is blood-purifying.

Ground nut oil is another name for **peanut oil** or monkey nut oil. It is used mainly for frying. These nuts often contain a fungus which has a cancer-producing effect.

Maize oil is another name for **corn oil.** It can be used in hot poultices, together with camphor, and applied to an inflamed area. Use 1 cup of maize oil with 50–100 crystals (about 20g). Shake well before use.

Medicinal oils – cardamom, cumin, cinnamon, clove and camphor oils (and many more) are all carminative – they relieve flatulence.

Mustard oil is a contra-irritant. It generates heat and is good news if you have inflammation of the skin. Mustard oil massage is often used as a strong stimulant in India before a bath. For hip pains, apply mustard oil to the hips and cover with bruised cabbage leaves. It is important to bruise the leaves sufficiently for the liquid to emerge. Two large leaves on the hip will help relieve the pain.

Olive oil – there are about 22 varieties available. Extra virgin oil is the best. See entry under Olives.

Poppy seed oil is good for soothing the nerves. It is tasty in salads.

Rapeseed oil is effective for inflammation of the joints, in the same way that mustard oil is. Only when purified is it edible. (In Spain, some 2000 people died when unpurified rapeseed oil was mixed with olive oil.) Unpurified rapeseed oil is used only as a machine lubricant.

Sesame oil is antifungal and anti-infectious. It is also anticancerous. When used in the nose it heals sinusitus by extracting the toxins. Place 2–3 drops in the nose before bedtime.

Vegetable oil is made from a mixture of different vegetables. Most vegetable oils are polyunsaturated.

Wheatgerm oil is very rich in vitamin E. It should be applied externally. Mixed with vitamin A and D, it combats skin diseases such as eczema and scrofulous. It will also heal scar tissue. **Caution**: wheatgerm oil can become rancid quite quickly.

Oil treatments

FOR ANAEMIA

Hazelnut, Brazil nut, walnut and *pumpkin seed oils* are very rich in zinc and can be useful for anaemia – when there is insufficient zinc in the blood, iron is not assimilated. Zinc B13 taken as a mineral substitute pill increases the blood's capacity to utilize iron.

TO LOWER BLOOD CHOLESTEROL

Drink 1 eggcup of *safflower, olive* or *sunflower oil* before going to bed. Safflower oil is the most effective.

TO RELIEVE CONSTIPATION

Castor and *olive oil* are both used for constipation.

FOR DETOXIFICATION

A good detoxifying effect can be achieved by swilling a 30ml mixture of *olive, sunflower* and *sesame oils* in your mouth until it froths, then spit it out. Frothing is a sign that toxins are being extracted. Most toxins return to the inner lining of the mouth, because the tongue is directly connected to the stomach. This treatment can therefore be a most successful means of extracting poisons from the system.

TO HEAL EAR PROBLEMS

Sesame oil and *almond oil* are both useful.

AS AN ENEMA

Mix 250ml of *olive* and *castor* oil with 1 teaspoon of bicarbonate of soda. This will soothe the intestinal muscles. Dissolve the soda in a little water before mixing with the oil. You will need to use a syringe since greater pressure is required with oil than with water or coffee because of its viscosity. Use a special rectal syringe, which is slightly bent. Lie on your left side so that the solution can enter the sigmoid (part of the descending colon) and gently rotate your body while lying down.

TO CONTROL HAEMORRHOIDS

Olive oil, or *castor oil* and lemon juice in equal proportions, can control haemorrhoids when injected into the rectum using a special syringe. Use 1 cup, making sure that the lemon is filtered. Since the mixture is strongly astringent, it will not travel far into the colon. Haemorrhoids are simply veins swollen with blood as a result of a collapsed valve. (Varicose veins are also veins with collapsed valves.)

FOR JOINT INFLAMMATION, ARTHRITIS

Maize, mustard, sesame, walnut, linseed, wheatgerm, castor and rapeseed oils are all good for fomentation (poultices). The strongest is mustard oil. Castor-oil packs draw out arthritic pains.

TO SOFTEN STAGNANT BLOOD

To soften stagnant blood after a thrombosis use *calendula oil* with some drops of the essential oil of *wintergreen*. The best wintergreen oil would probably have to be purchased from a veterinarian. Although used mainly for horses, it is most effective for arthritis, rheumatoid spondylitis and rheumatism.

✳ Olives

– richer in vitamin C than lemons

TASTE sweet
ELEMENT earth

Did you know?

Olives counteract poisoning from fish and mushrooms, relieve hangovers and help to dissolve bones after eating fish.

Olive oil only works as a remedy when cold-pressed. The best type is extra virgin olive oil. It is useful for lowering blood cholesterol.

Natural therapeutic values of olive oil

- cholagogic, demulcent, emollient, laxative, anticancerous, antioxidant, cathartic

❋ Onions

– combat colds and coughs; red onions contain large amounts of vitamins A and E

TASTE pungent
ELEMENT metal

Nutritional values
- rich in vitamins A and E, which are antioxidants. Oxidants are substances, like free radicals, that destroy the tissue.
- rich in vitamin C, calcium, iron (especially red onions) and sulphur

Did you know?
Onions constitute one of the most powerful remedies that can be commonly found in the average household. The healing effect of red onions is greater than that of white onions. While the white onion is rich in vitamin E, the red onion contains both vitamins A and E. The onion is a powerful healer not only when eaten raw, but also fried, dried or boiled.

The fresh juice of an onion can be rubbed on burns, bites and stings. Influenza patients, given the juice of pounded onions in a warm infusion 3 times a day at the onset of the disease, can often recover within 2–3 days. Fresh onion juice mixed with honey makes a good cough syrup.

Natural therapeutic effects
- antioxidant, antidiabetic, antifungal, antiviral, antibacterial, anticancerous, anthelmintic, antiseptic, antispasmodic, carminative, diuretic, expectorant, stomachic, tonic

Beneficial in the treatment of
- catarrh
- anaemia
- coughs and colds
- influenza
- liver cirrhosis
- dropsy
- kidney diseases
- tuberculosis
- germs in the mouth (chew raw onions for 3 minutes)

- ascites (abdominal dropsy)
- bronchitis
- insomnia
- jaundice
- splenic enlargement
- dyspepsia
- toothache
- bruises
- earache
- nervous debility
- brain fatigue
- anxiety
- heroine (morphine) and tobacco addiction

Onions also strenghten the lungs and cleanse the colon.

Prevention

Onions can help to prevent severe diseases of the respiratory system.

❋ Oranges

– strengthen the immune system; alkaline-forming

TASTE sour
ELEMENT wood

Nutritional values
- rich in mineral salts, especially calcium
- rich in vitamins, especially C

Beneficial in the treatment of
- fevers
- catarrh
- colds
- acidosis
- hyperacidity of the stomach

Did you know?

Oranges are strongly alkaline-forming. They are a good supplement for arthritics and meat eaters who need to combat acidosis. Grilled oranges are very strong immune strengtheners. The pith contains vitamin P (bioflavanoids) and the flesh is rich in vitamin C. Through the process of grilling, the pith and the fleshy part mingle, making it easier for the body to absorb the bioflavanoids and vitamin C. When vitamins C and P combine, they activate the immune system of the body and help it to eliminate toxins. A monofast with grilled oranges is a first step in the treatment of Aids, hepatitis C and B, herpes and non-specific urethritis. It can also be used to break down tumours. (See the Blood-Purifying Diet, p. 21.)

❋ Oysters

– blood builder, antidepressant, aphrodisiac; rich in zinc

TASTE salty
ELEMENT water

Nutritional value
* rich in zinc (especially smoked oysters!)
* rich in omega 3 fatty acids
* rich in tyrosine (amino-acid)

Did you know?

Oysters are one of the purest protein foods on earth. Tyrosine stimulates the brain to produce dopamine and norepinephrine, two neurotransmitters that mentally energize the brain and have an uplifting effect. The high zinc content of oysters makes them a strong aphrodisiac, especially for men. Zinc is needed to produce hormones and sperm. Omega 3 fatty acids – found in most seafoods – are known to lower the cholesterol, reduce the risk of all cardiac diseases and decrease arteriosclerosis. Their significance was discovered after it was observed that Eskimos have a very low incidence of heart disease.

Natural therapeutic effects
* blood-purifying, aphrodisiac

Oysters also work on the kidneys and blood and soften hard spots in the body.

Beneficial in the treatment of
- insomnia
- indecisiveness
- swellings of the abdomen
- hypertension
- rheumatoid arthritis
- asthma
- allergies
- psoriasis
- cancer
- zinc deficiencies
- eating disorders
- cardiac troubles

❈ Papaya

– contain papain and pepsin, enzymes which stimulate and aid digestion; cooked green papaya is effective for diarrhoea

TASTE sweet
ELEMENT earth

Nutritional value
- very rich in vitamin A, superior even to cod liver oil and butter
- rich in calcium
- strongly alkaline
- leaves contain carpaine, a heart stimulant

Did you know?
When you chew the black seeds of a ripe papaya, papain, a protein-digesting enzyme similar to pepsin, is released. The milky juice of dried papaya contains an even higher amount of papain, which is known to help with dyspepsia and intestinal irritation, and where there is deficiency of gastric juices or an excess of unhealthy mucus in the stomach.

The ripe fruit is used in cosmetics. Rubbed on the skin it can remove freckles and blemishes.

Natural therapeutic effects
- digestive, stomachic, vermifugic, vulnerary
- seeds – anthelmintic, carminative, emmenagogic

Beneficial in the treatment of
- flatulence
- liver troubles
- diarrhoea
- dyspepsia
- constipation

❋ Paprika

– very rich in vitamin C

TASTE hot
ELEMENT fire

Did you know?
Paprika is useful for opening the lungs and improving blood circulation.

❋ Parsley

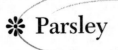

– good diuretic; stimulates blood flow through capillaries; blood purifier; should be taken moderately

TASTE pungent
ELEMENT metal

Did you know?
Parsley assists oxygen metabolism and helps to maintain the normal action of the adrenal and thyroid glands.

It is also good for the eyes and optic nerves. Mix raw parsley and carrot juice to treat weak eyes, lazy pupils, ulceration of the cornea, cataracts, conjunctivitis or ophthalmia.

Parsley effectively helps keep capillaries and arterioles in a good condition.

Natural therapeutic effects
- antispasmodic, carminative, diuretic, emmenagogic, expectorant

Beneficial in the treatment of
- problems of genito-urinary tract
- albuminuria   *see   140 + 146*
- nephritis and kidney troubles

It can also be used to counteract the smell of garlic in the mouth.

❋ Peaches

– very nutritious; rich in iron

TASTE sweet
ELEMENT earth

Nutritional values
- rich in iron
- alkaline

Beneficial in the treatment of
- anaemia
- indigestion
- dyspepsia
- chronic intestinal disorders
- blood impurities

MAGIC RECIPE FOR HAIR GROWTH
Bruise 4 kernels and boil in a cup of vinegar, then apply to the scalp. Whilst there is no known cure for baldness, this remedy is said to stimulate hair growth when the hair is thin.

✻ Pears

*– blood purifier; laxative – increase peristaltic movement of the
lower colon*

TASTE sweet
ELEMENT earth

Did you know?
Pears are reported to dissolve stones in the bladder. To achieve this result,
a monofast would be most effective.

Natural therapeutic effects
• alkaline-forming, laxative

✻ Peas

– blood-builder; have contraceptive powers

TASTE astringent
ELEMENT water

Nutritional values
• lower in protein than lentils or beans
• rich in chlorophyll

Did you know?
Garlic, ginger, cumin, oregano, asafoetida and lemon peel added to pea
soup will assist digestion and help to prevent wind.

   An Indian scientist, Dr Sanyal, observed that the population of Tibet
had remained stable for 200 years. He suspected that the reason for this
was something in their diet, which consisted mainly of barley and peas.
He eventually succeeded in identifying an antifertilizing chemical,
m-xylohydroquinone, in the pea. It appears to reduce fertility in women
and the sperm count in men by half.

RECIPE
Boil some fresh peas, drain, then break a raw egg over them. Put the lid

on again and and in a few minutes the steam will cook the egg. Serve with salt and freshly ground black pepper to taste. It is quite delicious.

✳ Peppercorns

– kill germs and bacteria; work instantly with sore throats and blocked nasal passages

TASTE pungent
ELEMENT metal

Did you know?
The outer skin is anticatarrhal. Powdered black pepper has usually had the outer skin removed, rendering it catarrh-producing. Eating coarse pepper reduces catarrh.

Natural therapeutic effects
* aromatic, stimulant, carminative, digestive, stomachic, nervine tonic, resolvent, cholagogic, diuretic, emmenagogic, antiperiodic

Beneficial in the treatment of
* catarrh
* sore throats
* colds with sneezing

REMEDY
Chew about 20 peppercorns and then drink a cup of hot water – you may well end up dancing but it will clear your throat and sinuses.

✳ Pineapples

– excellent for rheumatic complaints; remove uric acid from body

TASTE sweet
ELEMENT earth

Nutritional values
- contain bromelaine
- rich in chlorine
- contain malic acid

Did you know?
The enzyme bromelaine helps to digest meat, egg white, casein (a protein of milk), fish and beans. For dyspepsia, a glass of fresh pineapple juice relieves the problem. Chlorine removes waste products from the body by stimulating the kidney functions.

Natural therapeutic effects
- anti-arthritic, antirheumatic

Beneficial in the treatment of
- overworked kidneys
- oedema
- heart and kidney diseases
- dropsical swellings

Caution
Unripe pineapple can produce mouth ulcers.

✳ Plums and prunes

– cleanse the intestinal tract; laxative

TASTE sweet
ELEMENT earth

Nutritional value
- rich in calcium, phosphorus and iron
- rich in potassium
- source of vitamins A, B and C
- contain mainly malic acid, but also citric, tartaric, benzoic and boric acid
- contain small amounts of benzoic acid, which acidifies the urine

Did you know?
Sun-dried prunes have the advantage of drying without fermenting, unlike plums which ferment when sulphur-dried.

Prunes are famous as a laxative. They move the bowels quickly. Best results are obtained when they are soaked overnight and eaten in the morning.

Natural therapeutic effects
• anthelmintic, astringent, laxative

REMEDY
Plums and prunes work directly on the nervous system. They can be quite uplifting when you are feeling irritable. Make prune tea with 50g of dried prunes soaked overnight in 250ml of distilled water. Let it simmer until the prunes are soft. Strain and add lemon to taste.

Caution
Avoid prunes and plums if your bladder or kidneys are irritated, or if you already have an acidic condition such as acidosis, arthritis or gout – or if you eat a lot of meat.

Umeboshi (plums pickled in salt)

TASTE salty
ELEMENT water

Nutritional value
• rich in vitamin C

Did you know?
Umeboshis are a good aid to digestion.

Natural therapeutic effect
• anti-infective, carminative

❋ Pomegranates

– good for kidney troubles and fevers; astringent

TASTE sweet/sour
ELEMENT water

Nutritional value
• high tannin content (rind)

Did you know?
Pomegranates are best eaten in winter when the even more effective watermelons are not available. The seeds are a second-class diuretic – the sour, red pomegranate seeds are more helpful for healing, while those of the yellow/white pomegranates are too sweet and do not have much of an effect on the kidneys.

Use the rind to make tea to help with skin problems and mouth irritations, and as a gargle for the throat.

❋ Potatoes

– highly alkaline; work against arthritis and rheumatism; the raw juice is effective for stomach ulcers

TASTE sweet
ELEMENT earth

Nutritional values
• rich in alkaline salts such as sodium and potassium, but lacking in calcium (therefore needs to balanced with green vegetables)
• rich in vitamins A and B
• the skin is rich in chlorogenic acid which prevents cell mutation leading to cancer

Did you know?
The water in which potatoes are boiled contains about 60 per cent of the minerals and should not be thrown away. There is also much goodness in their skins. So see to it that you buy organically grown potatoes, cook

them in a way that will retain most of their vitamins, and eat the skins. They are best oven-baked in their jackets.

Raw potato is digestible only when the starch is removed. Grate the potato and squeeze out the starch by hand. Mixed with onions, tomatoes, lettuce and other raw vegetables it makes a most delicious salad.

Natural therapeutic effects
- anti-inflammatory, anti-ulcerous

Beneficial in the treatment of
- acidosis
- Bright's disease
- heart disease
- arteriosclerosis
- high blood pressure
- tooth decay
- cyclic vomiting
- rheumatism
- hardening of the arteries
- chronic constipation
- uric acid diseases and gout
- premature ageing
- intestinal toxaemia
- renal calculus
- re-storage of synovial fluid
- first-degree burns

Boiled potato peel is useful for prostate inflammation (make them into a pack) and a potato peel diet is very effective for arthritis (see Arthritis, p. 68).

Caution
Potatoes that have sprouted are poisonous. Throw them away. They contain solanin, which is harmful and should not be eaten. Potatoes should not be kept for too long and should not to be exposed to sunlight.

❋ Probiotics

– symbiotic with anabolic bacteria such as acidophilus *and* bifidus

There are approximately 400 species of bacteria living in the intestines. They make up about 1½kg of our body weight. One-third of faeces consists of bacteria. They work for us and in return we give them space in which to live: a veritable guest–host partnership.

Among the jobs they perform for us, they:

- aid digestion
- produce vitamin B
- digest milk and process milk calcium
- keep out unfriendly bacteria
- stimulate bowel movement
- control cholesterol levels
- eliminate toxins from radiation and pollution
- maintain the alkaline/acid balance
- control the growth of cancerous and tumour cells
- aid re-absorption of vitamins, enzymes and hormones via the large intestines

Bacteria in symbiosis with the intestinal environment form the immune system. When we upset this balance we create space for unfriendly bacteria such as *candida albicans, E. coli* and *staphylococcus*.

Changes in our intestinal flora can cause:

- constipation
- the destruction of friendly bacteria – through the use of drugs, especially antibiotics
- imbalance to the alkaline-acid balance in the body – through reduced production of acid in the stomach (dyspepsia)
- stress

Meat-processing bacteria are aerobic. These bacteria grow in an environment where oxygen is available. They need meat and fats. When we eat excessive amounts of meat, aerobic bacteria colonize our intestines and reduce the volume of anaerobic (friendly) bacteria. Friendly bacteria such as *Lactobacillus acidophilus, L. bulgaricus*, and *Bifidobacterium* need an oxygen-free alkaline environment in which to grow.

Bioyoghurt

TASTE sweet and sour
ELEMENT earth and wood

Nutritional value
• rich in calcium

Bioyoghurt contains intestine-friendly *acidophilus* bacteria. It is most effective when eaten with banana. This prevents the enzymes and bacteria from being destroyed by the gastric juices and hydrochloric acid before they reach the intestines.

Beneficial in the treatment of
• duodenal and gastric ulcers
• mucus colitis

Bioyoghurt is also useful to restore colon-friendly bacteria after the use of antibiotics.

❋ Psyllium seed husks

– colon cleanser and laxative

TASTE sweet
ELEMENT earth

Did you know?
Psyllium husks are the most popular fibre for cleansing the colon. They are found in many ready-made products. Eat them in combination with fenugreek powder and slippery elm (see Constipation, p. 82).

Natural therapeutic effect
• laxative

Beneficial in the treatment of
• constipation
• excess weight

Psyllium husks are also useful as a colon cleanser (they remove metallic toxins) and stool softener.

❋ Pumpkins

– rich in beta carotene; eye strengthener and lung protector

TASTE sweet
ELEMENT earth

Nutritional value
- contain vitamins A, B and C
- rich in iron and zinc

Did you know?
The more orange the pumpkin, the better. Orange is the colour of beta carotene, the factor that is needed to produce vitamin A. This is the vitamin that you need to lower the risk of lung disease. Together with carrots, pumpkin is good food for smokers.

When chewed in the evening, the seeds combat tapeworms. Eat about 100 with sugar before bedtime, followed by 1 tablespoon of castor oil the next morning.

Natural therapeutic effects
- pulp – alkaline-forming, eye-strengthening, anti-infective, antioxidant, blood-building
- seeds – laxative, purgative

❋ Radishes

– rich in sulphur: red, black and white

TASTE pungent
ELEMENT metal

Nutritional value
- rich in iron, calcium, sodium

Natural therapeutic effects
- antispasmodic, astringent, cholagogic, diuretic
- seeds – laxative, diuretic and lithontriptic, emmenagogic

Beneficial in the treatment of
- tuberculosis
- anaemia
- disorders of the nervous system
- coughs
- rheumatism
- gall bladder problems
- chronic bronchitis
- flatulence
- diarrhoea
- headaches
- insomnia

Radish seeds are useful to reduce heavy menstrual flow.

REMEDY

The juice of 150g of fresh radishes in the morning and evening relieves piles. Or, for a 3-week juice cure, take 100ml before breakfast each day, gradually increasing to 350ml over 2 weeks. Then reduce the quantity back to 100ml over the following week.

❇ Raspberries

– strengthen the immune system; help with rheumatism

TASTE sour
ELEMENT wood

Nutritional value
- highly alkaline
- rich in iron
- contain vitamin C

Natural therapeutic effects
- anti-emetic, astringent, laxative

Beneficial in the treatment of
- fevers

- rheumatism
- pains in joints and limbs

Raspberry leaves

The leaves are rich in vitamins, calcium, phosphorus and iron – and an unknown factor that helps to prevent miscarriages (make a tea from the leaves and drink every morning); it also promotes less painful labour.

Beneficial in the treatment of
- diarrhoea
- dysentery
- passive haemorrhage from the stomach

✳ Rice

– lowers high blood pressure

TASTE astringent
ELEMENT metal

Nutritional value
- rich in vitamin B (if the husk is not removed)
- low in proteins, low in salts and calcium (the least acid-forming grain)

A rice diet is beneficial in the treatment of
- renal disorders
- hypertensive vascular disease
- high blood pressure

Other uses
- as an enema for bowel afflictions
- use rice water for the treatment of gastric and duodenal ulcers
- use rice bran for hypercalcuria
- use rice flour to make a poultice for measles, inflammations of the skin, burns, heat and irritations, or to apply to an abscess, boils, ulcers, inflamed piles

✳ Rosemary

– stimulates the blood circulation

TASTE bitter
ELEMENT fire

Natural therapeutic effects
- antispasmodic, cholagogic, emmenagogic, stimulant, stomachic
- preservative (in sausages)

Beneficial in the treatment of
- poor circulation
- low blood pressure
- dandruff – use shampoo with rosemary (stimulates the circulation of the skin)
- hypertension (tea is soothing)

Rosemary also helps to promote liver function.

The leaves cooked in wine, or a salve made from rosemary oil is beneficial in the treatment of
- rheumatism
- scrofulous sores
- eczema
- bruises
- wounds

RECIPE
Rosemary tea is useful as a mouthwash to counteract halitosis. Steep 1 teaspoon of dried flowering tops or leaves in ½ cup of water. Take up to 1 cup a day.

Caution
Excessive amounts of rosemary taken internally can cause fatal poisoning.

❄ Sage (red and green)

— soothes sore throats; reduces night-sweats; cleans the teeth

TASTE bitter
ELEMENT fire

Natural therapeutic effects
- antihydrotic, antispasmodic, astringent

Beneficial in the treatment of
- nervous conditions
- trembling
- depression
- vertigo
- diarrhoea, gastritis, enteritis
- mucous congestion in the respiratory passages and the stomach

Other uses
- gargle with tea when you have a sore throat
- rub the crushed leaves on the teeth to whiten them
- drink tea to reduce perspiration (eg night-sweats)
- use crushed fresh sage leaves as first aid for insect bites

RECIPE
To make sage tea, steep 1 teaspoon of leaves in ½ cup of hot water for 30 minutes. Drink 1 cup a day, 1 tablespoon at a time.

Caution
Extended or excessive use of sage can cause symptoms of poisoning.

❄ Salt

— essential for all human beings

ELEMENT water

Natural therapeutic effects
- antiseptic, emetic

Did you know?

Sodium is contained in salt, and in the body it is carried in the blood. Sodium regulates all thermostatic functions. It is most unhealthy to eat too many vegetables with an insufficient quantity of salt. Rocksalt is better than table salt. Seasalt, which is not purified and iodinized, is healthy in reasonable quantities.

✳ Sardines

– rich in iron

TASTE astringent
ELEMENT fire

Did you know?

When you use sardines out of a tin, it is better to drain off the oil and replace it with lemon juice. For benefits, see Mackerel, p. 188.

✳ Seaweed

good or bad?

– highly alkalizing; lowers high blood pressure and LDL (low density lipoprotein) cholesterol

TASTE salty
ELEMENT water

Nutritional value
• very rich in calcium
• highly alkaline-forming

Did you know?

Nori, kelp, laminaria, kombu, chlorella, wakame, hiziki, Irish moss and Welsh Larnalnead are all types of seaweed.

Natural therapeutic effects
• anticancerous, antitumorous, anticoagulant, anti-ulcerous, antibacterial

Beneficial in the treatment of
- high blood pressure
- high blood cholesterol

❋ Seeds

– pumpkin, black and white sesame, sunflower

TASTE sweet
ELEMENT earth

Nutritional value

Sunflower, pumpkin and sesame seeds are excellent sources of protein, essential fatty acids, vitamins, minerals and trace elements. They are particularly rich in magnesium and calcium.

Pumpkin seeds are rich in vitamin B, phosphorus, iron and zinc. For prostate troubles, eat 50g a day for 3 months.

White sesame seeds are rich in calcium and vitamin E, and have aphrodisiac qualities. During pregnancy and lactation, take at least 30g to supplement calcium needs.

Black sesame seeds are exceptionally rich in iron and useful for anaemic people. If you bruise easily, take 50g a day for 3 months. Use red and black varieties with their skin.

Sunflower seeds contain vitamin E, B complex, iron, magnesium and zinc.

❋ Slippery elm

– soothes the intestinal tract

TASTE bland
ELEMENT wood

Did you know?

The inner bark is used as tea or powder. It is slippery and soothing.

Natural therapeutic values
- demulcent, diuretic, emollient

Beneficial in the treatment of
- sore throats
- diarrhoea
- dysentery
- urinary problems
- inflamed and irritated skin – use externally
- wounds

✻ Spinach

– blood builder; lung protector; eye-strengthener

TASTE sweet
ELEMENT earth

Nutritional value
- rich in zinc, calcium, iron, manganese, copper and iodine, chlorophyll
- richest source of vitamin A
- contains vitamins B, C and D
- alkaline

Did you know?
Spinach came to be viewed as a cure for iron deficiency with extraordinary effect due to a mistake in notation. The Popeye legend was born when spinach was mistakenly noted as containing 0.1g of iron instead of 0.001g. Raw spinach contains a small amount of oxalic acid which can be removed with parboiling.

Natural therapeutic effects
- haemoglobin-building, alkaline-forming

Spinach juice is beneficial in the treatment of
- night-blindness
- bleeding gums
- pyorrhoea

- duodenal ulcers
- constipation
- gout
- abscesses and boils
- glandular disturbances
- obesity
- high or low blood pressure
- swellings of the legs and ankles
- rheumatism
- eye diseases
- nervous exhaustion and migraine
- sore throats – use as a gargle

Spinach is also good for improving the eyesight in general.

✳ Strawberries

– useful for gout and rheumatic problems

TASTE sour
ELEMENT wood

Nutritional value
- contain mainly citric acid and malic acid
- have large amounts of kalium (5 times more than bananas – only figs, dates and other dried fruits are richer in kalium)
- very rich in vitamins A and C (to combat the formation of uric acid)
- rich in iron (richer than most vegetables, such as onions, beets, carrots, radishes and potatoes)
- super-rich in pectin

Natural therapeutic effects
- fruit – antiviral, anticancerous
- leaf tea – alkalizing, blood-cleansing

Beneficial in the treatment of
- gout
- rheumatism

✳ Sugar cane

– very good for blood pressure

TASTE sweet
ELEMENT earth

Nutritional value
• juice – rich in iron, calcium, manganese

Did you know?
Sugar cane is a good antidote against poisoning by copper and arsenic.

Molasses is very rich in iron and calcium and can be directly assimilated by the body.

✳ Sulphur

– blood purifier; present in all cruciferous vegetables

TASTE pungent
ELEMENT fire

Sulphur-containing foods include dried soya beans, kidney beans, peanuts, oats, Brazil nuts, dried peas, parsley, wheat, almonds, watercress, broccoli, barley, pecans, rice, cauliflowers, dried coconut, dried figs, onions, cabbages, dates, asparagus, avocados, okra, radishes.

Among sulphur-containing plants, herbs and spices are asafoetida, chervil, dill, endive, fennel, garlic, nettles, sage, sesame seeds, sunflower seeds and thyme.

Did you know?
Many dried fruits are preserved with sulphur. In small amounts it expels toxins. Large amounts are not well received by the body. Sulphur can be cleaned from dried fruit in the following way. Add 4 teaspoons of hydrogen peroxide to 250ml of water. Leave the dried fruit in this solution for 5 minutes. The sulphur will be converted into a gas. The same solution can be used for 4–5 washings.

Sulphur is also involved in bone growth, blood clotting and muscle metabolism.

❋ Swedes

– rich in calcium

TASTE sweet
ELEMENT earth

Nutritional value
• rich in calcium and iron

Did you know?
Swedes constitute a tasty and filling dish when cooked and mashed with potatoes or turnips.

❋ Tea tree oil

– highly anti-infectious; anti-inflammatory; antiseptic

TASTE bitter
SMELL stringent
ELEMENT metal

Did you know?
The oil is very effective for inhalation when the nasal passages are blocked. It is also helpful when rubbed into sore muscles, when diluted with other oils.

❋ Thuja

– combats viral infections from clamydia to warts; detoxifies

SMELL astringent
ELEMENT metal

Natural therapeutic effects
• diaphoretic, emmenagogic

Used internally, thuja is beneficial in the treatment of
- muscular aches
- rheumatism

It can also expel toxins.

Used externally, it is useful for
- warts
- rheumatic pains
- skin problems

Thuja can also be taken as a tea to relieve headaches and to reduce swellings and heart pain.

❋ Thyme

– releases mucus from respiratory system; relaxes digestive tract

TASTE bitter
ELEMENT fire

Natural therapeutic effects
- anthelmintic, antispasmodic, carminative, diaphoretic, expectorant, sedative

Beneficial in the treatment of
- throat and bronchial problems
- gastro-intestinal problems

Caution
Excessive use of thyme is poisonous and leads to overstimulation of the thyroid gland.

❋ Tomatoes

– very rich in magnesium

TASTE sour
ELEMENT wood

Nutritional value
- very rich in vitamins A, B and C
- rich in minerals, especially magnesium
- rich in iron (contain twice as much as milk does)

Natural therapeutic effects (on the blood)
- alkalizing, cleansing

Beneficial in the treatment of
- acidosis
- premature ageing
- torpid liver
- atonic dyspepsia
- biliousness
- bronchitis and asthma
- poisons in the body

Tomatoes also act as a kidney tonic.

❋ Turmeric

TASTE bitter
ELEMENT metal

Natural therapeutic effects
- blood-purifying, tonic, carminative, diuretic, appetizing, aphrodisiac, antiseptic, anticancerous

Beneficial in the treatment of
- piles
- biliousness
- diseases of the blood
- bronchitis
- ophthalmia
- diarrhoea
- lumbago
- gonorrhoea
- pain in the joints

- tonsillitis
- boils and carbuncles

❋ Turnips

– very rich in sulphur

TASTE sweet
ELEMENT earth

Nutritional value
- high in sulphur
- rich in vitamin C, calcium
- leaves – rich in vitamins A and C, calcium, iron and chlorophyll

Did you know?
Turnip juice is useful for hardening soft bones, alkalizing and purifying the blood, hardening teeth, and for diseases of the respiratory system.

❋ Vine leaves

– diuretic; dissolve kidney stones

TASTE sweet
ELEMENT earth

Did you know?
Vine leaves are much used in the cuisine of the Middle East, Greece and Turkey. Vine leaves stuffed with rice help with constipation, and used as tea they can dissolve calcium deposits in the kidneys. In combination with watermelon they can dissolve kidney stones.

Natural therapeutic effects
- cathartic, diuretic

Beneficial in the treatment of
- kidney stones
- constipation

✳ Walnuts

— very rich in zinc; the bark of the tree is used to treat paradontosis and other gum problems

TASTE sweet
ELEMENT earth

Because walnuts contain large amounts of protein, they are a valuable supplement for brain workers (see Brain Fatigue diet, p. 52).

Walnut tree bark

Natural therapeutic effects
• astringent, anthelmintic, detergent, lactifugic

Did you know?
Walnut bark is used to strengthen the gums and to stop mammary secretion, as a gargle for sore throats, and as a bath additive for rheumatism, gout, glandular swelling, sweaty feet, acne, dandruff and other skin problems.

Walnut kernels

Natural therapeutic effect
• aphrodisiac

Beneficial in the treatment of
• heartburn
• colic
• dysentery

Walnut oil

Natural therapeutic effects
• mild laxative, cholagogic, anthelmintic

Especially beneficial in the treatment of
• tapeworms

❇ Water

Human beings comprise 80 per cent water, and it is also our most abiding requirement. When we are either too alkaline or too acidic, our bodies retain water in order to dilute the toxins and prevent problems resulting from the imbalance.

Salty water is antiseptic.

❇ Watercress

– diuretic; blood builder; cleanses the respiratory system

TASTE pungent
ELEMENT metal

Nutritional value
- rich in iron, phosphates, potassium,
- contains a considerable amount of iodine and sulphur
- high in vitamins A and C

Did you know?
Bruised leaves are said to be able to remove pimples and freckles.

Natural therapeutic effects
- diuretic, expectorant, purgative, stimulant, stomachic – can also work as a psychic stimulant

Beneficial in the treatment of
- headaches
- biliousness
- asthma
- coughs with expectoration
- sleeplessness

Watercress seeds have special healing powers to combat
- hiccups
- indigestion
- diarrhoea

- general debility
- flatulence
- seminal debility
- leucorrhoea

Caution

Watercress must be washed very thoroughly before being consumed.

❀ Watermelons

– best remedy for all kidney problems; diuretic

TASTE sweet
ELEMENT earth

Nutritional value
- rich in vitamins A, B and C
- contains many minerals
- contains no proteins – except in the seeds

Natural therapeutic effects
- diuretic – the only fruit that can affect many different kidney ailments
- the seeds, when dried and roasted, lower the blood pressure

REMEDY

A watermelon juice fast will remove kidney stones. Continue until the kidney stones are gone. Take 5 litres of juice (without seeds) and boil down to 2½ litres. Drink this and no other liquids for 7–21 days.

❀ White willow bark

– contains salicylic acid (a pain killer); prevents blood from
  clotting

TASTE bitter
ELEMENT fire

Did you know?

White willow bark is the source from which aspirin was originally derived. It contains salicin, which is converted into salicylic acid in the body. Aspirin is now made from synthetically produced salicylic acid.

Salicylic acid also prevents the blood from clotting and is used after strokes and for heart disease. A cup of white willow bark tea can have the same effect. The tea also contains other substances (minerals and vitamins) which balance each other.

Natural therapeutic effects

• anodyne, antiseptic, astringent, diaphoretic, diuretic, febrifugic, tonic

White willow bark has the same effect as aspirin and is useful to counteract

• pain
• rheumatism
• fever
• gout and rheumatic problems – as a diuretic
• heartburn
• stomach ailments

❈ Wintergreen

– anaesthetic; used for pain in the joints

TASTE bitter
ELEMENT fire

Did you know?

Wintergreen oil is used for medicinal purposes. It contains methyl salicylate which is used to relieve pain, headaches and inflammations.

It relieves rheumatic pains in the joints when applied externally, and can be used as a douche for leucorrhoea. Make a tea with the leaves to gargle with when you have a sore throat or mouth.

Natural therapeutic effects

• analgesic, astringent, carminative, diuretic, stimulant

Caution
The oil should not be applied to the skin without first being diluted. It will otherwise cause irritation and can be poisonous.

❋ Yams (sweet potatoes)

– high in beta carotene, thus support eye and lung functions

TASTE sweet
ELEMENT earth

Nutritional value
• rich in beta carotene (the more yellow they are, the higher their beta carotene content

Did you know?
Recent research suggests that eating yams may increase the possibility of giving birh to twins. The theory is described in *The Food Pharmacy* by Jean Carper. Yams are rich in hormone-like substances that trigger the release of other hormones, including FSH (follicle-stimulating hormone). FSH is thought to stimulate the ovaries to release more than one ovum, setting the stage for multiple conception.

Yams also strengthen the spleen, lungs and kidneys and heat up the body.

Beneficial in the treatment of
• pre-menstrual syndrome
• diarrhoea
• coughs
• asthma
• chronic kidney disease
• diabetes
• seminal emission
• vaginal discharge

APPENDICES